Meals in Minutes

cookbook

ALSO BY THE AMERICAN HEART ASSOCIATION

The New American Heart Association Cookbook, 25th Anniversary Edition

American Heart Association Low-Fat, Low-Cholesterol Cookbook, Second Edition

American Heart Association Low-Salt Cookbook, Second Edition

American Heart Association Quick & Easy Cookbook

American Heart Association Around the World Cookbook

American Heart Association Low-Fat & Luscious Desserts

American Heart Association Kids' Cookbook

American Heart Association Guide to Heart Attack Treatment, Recovery, and Prevention

American Heart Association Family Guide to Stroke Treatment, Recovery, and Prevention

Living Well, Staying Well: The Ultimate Guide to Help Prevent Heart Disease and Cancer (with the American Cancer Society)

American Heart Association To Your Health! A Guide to Heart-Smart Living

American Heart Association 6 Weeks to Get Out the Fat

American Heart Association Fitting in Fitness

American Heart Association 365 Ways to Get Out the Fat

American Heart Association Brand-Name Fat and Cholesterol Counter, Second Edition

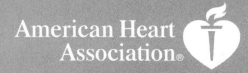

American Heart
Association®

Fighting Heart Disease and Stroke

Meals in
Minutes
cookbook

ver 200 all-new quick and easy low-fat recipes

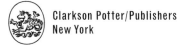

Clarkson Potter/Publishers
New York

Your contribution to the American Heart Association supports research
that helps make publications like this possible. For more information, call
1-800-AHA-USA1 (1-800-242-8721) or contact us online at www.
americanheart.org.

Published by Clarkson Potter/Publishers. Member of the Crown Publishing
Group, a division of Random House, Inc.
www.randomhouse.com

CLARKSON N. POTTER, POTTER, and colophon are registered trade-
marks of Random House, Inc.

Originally published in slightly different form in hardcover in 2000.

Printed in the United States of America.

Art direction by Naomi Osnos
Book design by Maura Fadden Rosenthal/MSpace
Illustrations by Ed Lam

Library of Congress Cataloging-in-Publication data is available on request.

ISBN 0-609-80977-6

10 9 8 7 6

First Paperback Edition

Front cover: Chicken Fajita Pasta with Chipotle Alfredo Sauce, page 165.
Photograph by Susan Goldman.

Preface

Sharing healthful, homemade meals and interesting conversation is a fading ritual, too often replaced by takeout and television or a slice of pizza and a dash out the door. You lead a hectic life, and mealtime often suffers.

However, you hold in your hands a book created to both nourish your body and respect your busy schedule. It shows you how to create wonderful dishes without a lot of fuss and bother.

And we didn't sacrifice a bit of flavor. All our recipes—from main dishes to sides to desserts—are a treat for your taste buds. Our recipes will show you how to have it all—delicious food that's good for you and that you can easily prepare in just minutes.

Welcome to a whole new world of reality cooking!

Acknowledgments

American Heart Association Science Consultant: Terry Bazzarre, Ph.D.

American Heart Association Managing Editor: Jane Anneken Ruehl

American Heart Association Senior Editor: Janice Roth Moss

American Heart Association Editor: Ann Melugin Williams

American Heart Association Editorial Assistant: Roberta Westcott Sullivan

Recipe Developers: Carol Ritchie
                     Nancy S. Hughes
                     Sarah Fritschner
                     DeeDee Stovel
                     Frank Criscuolo
                     Claire Criscuolo
                     George Geary

Writer: Cris Beam

Nutrient Analyses: Nutrition & Food Associates, Inc.

Contents

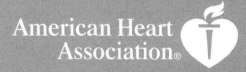

American Heart
Association®

Fighting Heart Disease and Stroke

Meals in
Minutes
cookbook

Introduction

Imagine that you can make small changes, minor adjustments, that can help you feel better and prevent or postpone major diseases. You'd jump at the chance, wouldn't you? Well, here's your opportunity—and it has to do with the next morsel you put in your mouth. What you eat has a big impact on your health, and luckily, you have control over your eating habits each and every day.

Sometimes, though, you'll need a little help, a little inspiration to keep from blowing your nutrition plan and running to the nearest take-out window. That's why we created this book—to spark your desire to be in the kitchen, preparing heart-healthy foods you'll crave again and again. We want you to dance into your nineties and hold your grand-children and great-grandchildren on your lap. And we want you to love every meal it took to get there.

Healthful food doesn't have to be bland or look as though it was prepared for a rabbit. Healthful food can be luscious, rich, and surprising. Healthful food can be Italian Quiche in Phyllo Shells, Spanish Shrimp, Sun-Dried Tomato Pesto Chicken and Pasta, or Lemon Cake with Apricot Glaze. As all the recipes in this book will prove, healthful food can be low in total fat, saturated fat, and cholesterol and moderate in sodium—and still look appealing and taste great. Also, healthful food can help protect you from the number one killer in this country, coronary heart disease.

A Changing Diet for Changing Times

The recipes in this book are more than just healthful and delicious—they are pretty speedy too. The tradition of a stay-at-home parent and seven nights a week of homemade, sit-down dinners has long been abandoned. Many of us are working longer hours at our jobs. At last count, about 72 percent of all women raising children also are working outside the home. About 78 percent of couples both work outside the home, so who has time to cook? Unfortunately, too many of us stuff down a large burger, fries, and a soda and call ourselves fed. Is it really possible to make the time for cooking and family conversation?

Yes.

No recipe in this book, whether it's an appetizer, a dessert, or a main dish, takes more than 20 minutes to prepare, so you'll have plenty of energy to truly share the meal you've made. We've even accounted for the fact that you don't like to plan. (According to a recent survey, most people don't know what they're going to have for dinner until about 4 P.M. that day.) You can make many of the dishes with ingredients you probably already have on hand—no stress, no extra trips to the store, no more heartache. Literally.

So, even though Americans are busier than ever and family structures continue to change, let's revive the custom of eating as a pleasure rather than as a distraction. Let's view cooking as creative and fun, rather than as a chore. It's all possible, with recipes as quick and easy as these.

Basics of a Healthful Diet

When you eat healthful, nutritious foods, you are rewarded with a better balance of all the essential nutrients, a diet low in saturated fat and cholesterol, and maybe even a cleaner bill of health.

On the other hand, when you eat poorly, you can raise your blood cholesterol levels and put yourself at risk for heart and blood vessel disease. One of the best gifts you can give yourself is to eat nourishing, vitamin-rich (and delicious!) meals and reduce your intake of fat and cholesterol.

Seven Steps to Good Nutrition

So what path do you take? To keep it simple, the American Heart Association has developed some basic dietary guidelines to reduce blood cholesterol and prevent or control high blood pressure.

1. Eat at least six servings of grain products and starchy vegetables daily.
2. Eat at least five servings of fruits and vegetables daily. Include at least one serving of citrus fruit or a vegetable high in vitamin C and one serving of a dark green, leafy vegetable or deep yellow vegetable.
3. Eat no more than 6 ounces (cooked weight) of lean meat, seafood, or skinless poultry per day. Have at least two servings of fish per week.
4. Include two or more servings of fat-free and low-fat dairy products daily if you are an adult. Children and adolescents should have three to four servings.
5. Choose a diet low in saturated fat, trans fat, and cholesterol and moderate in salt (sodium) and sugar. Eat no more than 10 percent of your calories as saturated fat. Limit yourself to less than 300 mg of cholesterol and less than 2,400 mg of sodium daily.
6. If you drink, limit yourself to one drink per day if you are a woman and two drinks per day if you are a man.

7. Balance food intake with physical activity to achieve and maintain a healthful weight.

A Cautionary Tale

"All things in moderation" is a great motto to remember when filling your plate. You shouldn't avoid all life's tasteful pleasures, but you should be especially mindful of the foods that may do the most harm. Here are the biggies to watch out for.

Fats

Diets high in fat, especially saturated fat and cholesterol, have been linked to heart disease, breast cancer, diabetes, and other troubles that can stem from obesity. It may take many years for these conditions to develop, but the way you feel after eating a high-fat meal—overfull, low energy—should give you a clue that your body doesn't like a lot of fat. You usually feel "lighter" and more energetic after eating a lower-fat meal—partly because high-fat meals take longer to digest.

To keep your heart and blood vessels at a healthy level, the American Heart Association recommends getting no more than 10 percent of your calories from saturated fat. If you have high cholesterol or coronary heart disease, the amount from saturated fat should be 7 percent or less.

The three basic types of fat are saturated, polyunsaturated, and monounsaturated. Saturated is the worst for you, because it raises blood cholesterol more than anything else you eat. Saturated fats are found in foods that come from animals. These foods include fatty meats, poultry with skin, whole milk, cheese, and butter, as well as in a few plant products—coconut, palm, and palm kernel oils. Polyunsaturated fats come from foods such as walnuts, corn oil, safflower oil, and fish. Monounsaturated fats, which are probably the least damaging, are predominant in olives, olive oil, canola oil, peanut oil, and avocados.

When you can pick between fats, avoid the saturated ones as much as possible. For example, butter and margarine both derive their calories from fat, but butter is loaded with the saturated kind. Therefore, margarine is the better choice. When it's hydrogenated and made firm, margarine also contains undesirable trans fatty acids. That's why we suggest buying the softer spreads with no more than 2 grams of saturated fat per tablespoon and with a liquid vegetable oil listed as the first ingredient.

Fatty foods are tempting, and sometimes you have to give in. That's okay. If you splurge on one meal or even one day, you can make it up the next. If you're trying to lose weight or maintain your weight, be sure that over the course of a week your calories from fat add up to 30 percent or less of your total calories, with no more than 10 percent from saturated fat.

To estimate the percentage of fat calories you take in, you need to know your total calories and the number of grams of fat you eat. Unless you are on a weight-loss program, you're probably not going to keep a record of what you eat every day. Here is a quick, easy way to figure how you're doing.

Count up the calories you eat in a typical day. Let's say you're a typical man who takes in 2,000 calories a day. (If you're a typical woman, you eat about 1,600 calories a day.) You also keep track of the number of grams of fat you eat in that same typical day. This is pretty easy to do with the nutrition labels on packaged foods and fresh meats and poultry. Fresh fruits and vegetables probably don't have a label. Except for avocados and coconuts, count them as zero fat. (But you do have to count added oil, margarine, and salad dressings.)

Say you counted 60 grams of fat on your typical day. Each gram of fat contains 9 calories, so you had $60 \times 9 = 540$ fat calories that day. Divide 540 by 2,000 (your total calories for the day) and multiply by 100 to get the percentage of fat calories: 27 percent. That's great!

You can eat a little more fat one day of the same week and still have a good average.

Cholesterol

Your body produces all the cholesterol it needs. In fact, cholesterol is found in every cell in your body. Cholesterol forms cell membranes, as well as some hormones. When you eat foods of animal origin (plants don't contain cholesterol), you take in extra cholesterol. It begins to build up on the artery walls and, together with cholesterol made from dietary fat, can lead to a heart attack. The American Heart Association recommends eating no more than 300 milligrams of cholesterol per day. You can keep your dietary cholesterol low by limiting your intake of meat and whole-milk dairy products, which are also high in saturated fat.

Cholesterol is most concentrated in organ meats, animal fat, and egg yolks. Try to skip the organ meats altogether, opt for fats that don't come from animals, and limit your egg yolk intake, including the yolks found in prepared foods such as many breads and noodles. Egg whites don't contain cholesterol, so eat as many of these as you please. When cooking, you can replace one whole egg with either two egg whites or egg substitute.

Alcohol

If you don't drink now, don't start. If you do drink, talk with your doctor about what amount is right for you. The American Heart Association recommends no more than one drink per day for women, two for men. Drinking more increases your risk for a number of health problems, including high blood pressure, stroke, liver problems, breast cancer, and possibly alcoholism.

Sodium

People tend to think of it as a bad word, but sodium helps the body maintain its delicate balance of fluids. The American Heart Association recommends no more than 2,400 milligrams (2.4 grams) of sodium per day for most people. This translates to about 1 teaspoon of salt (sodium chloride). If you have high blood pressure or there's a history of it in your family, however, your doctor may suggest a lower level. You can also help lower your blood pressure by following an active lifestyle, managing your weight, and eating plenty of fruit, vegetables, and non-fat or low-fat dairy products.

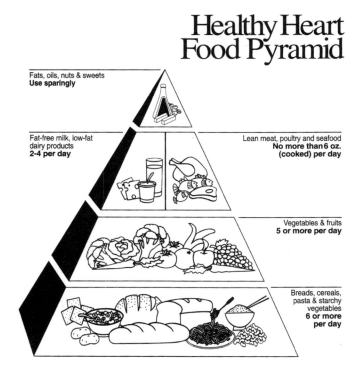

Healthy Heart Food Pyramid

Fats, oils, nuts & sweets
Use sparingly

Fat-free milk, low-fat dairy products
2-4 per day

Lean meat, poultry and seafood
No more than 6 oz. (cooked) per day

Vegetables & fruits
5 or more per day

Breads, cereals, pasta & starchy vegetables
6 or more per day

The Healthy Heart Food Pyramid

Visualize the food you eat on an average day. If you stack it all up by type, it should look like a pyramid, with starchy carbohydrates (breads, cereals, pasta, and beans) comprising the bulk of your diet, moving up through fruits and vegetables, then to nonfat and low-fat dairy products and meats, and finally, to a tiny bit of fats and oils at the tip. If you use this visual as a guide, your eating will be in line with American Heart Association recommendations.

Breads, Cereals, Pasta, and Starchy Vegetables

Every person over the age of two should have at least six servings of these carbohydrates each day. (A serving equals 1 slice of bread, ½ cup of hot cereal, 1 cup of flaked cereal, or 1 cup of cooked rice or pasta.) Foods from this foundation block of the pyramid should make up about 50 percent of the day's total calories. Select whole-grain breads instead of the less nutritious white breads, and don't forget those fiber-rich potatoes.

Vegetables and Fruits

A healthy person over the age of two should eat five or more servings of vegetables and fruits every day. Try to include at least one citrus fruit or a vegetable high in vitamin C and one serving of dark green, leafy vegetables. (A serving is one piece or ½ cup of fruit, ¾ cup of fruit or vegetable juice, 1 cup of a leafy or raw vegetable, or ½ cup of a cooked vegetable.)

Fat-Free (Skim) Milk and Nonfat and Low-Fat Dairy Products

Adults should have two to four servings of dairy products daily. Bump this to three to four servings for children and adolescents. (A serving equals 1 cup of fat-free milk, 1 cup of fat-free or low-fat yogurt, or 1 ounce of fat-free or reduced-fat cheese with fewer than 3 grams of fat.)

Lean Meat, Poultry, and Seafood

Foods in this part of the pyramid are great sources of protein and other essential nutrients, but they also contain fat. That's why we suggest no more than 6 ounces of cooked meat, poultry, or seafood a day. (A 3-ounce portion is about as big as a deck of cards. Four ounces of raw meat cooks down to about 3 ounces.) Don't worry about being protein deprived; most Americans already eat twice as much protein as they really need. In fact, it's a good idea to substitute dried beans, lentils, or tofu for the meat in your meal a few times a week.

Fats, Oils, Nuts, and Sweets

At the top of the pyramid are fats, oils, nuts, and sweets. Use these now-and-then foods sparingly. Aim for a daily intake of 5 to 8 teaspoons of polyunsaturated and monounsaturated fats and oils. In addition to counting margarine and cooking oil, include salad dressing and the fats in prepared foods in calculating your intake.

Other Considerations for a Healthy Heart

When planning your meals for the week, you will, of course, build in the foods your senses love. Remember, too, to plan on what your body loves. Here are a few things you can use liberally to help your system function at optimum levels.

Water

Don't forget! Good foods aren't the only things that your body needs. You also need water to carry nutrients to the cells. Experts suggest six to eight 8-ounce glasses of water every day.

Omega-3 Fatty Acids

Studies show that people who eat at least two servings of fish each week have a lower mortality rate from coronary heart disease than people who eat none. Why? Because fish—especially mackerel, coho and Atlantic salmon, carp, halibut, and herring—are high in omega-3 fatty acids. These substances help lower triglycerides, or blood fat, and may help reduce the risk for heart disease. So eat more fish!

If seafood isn't your thing, you can also find omega-3's in leafy green vegetables and soybeans, as well as in flaxseed oil, canola oil, walnuts, and walnut oil.

Fiber

Your grandmother probably called it "roughage" when she tried to get you to eat your broccoli or prunes. She was referring to fiber, which comes from the indigestible components of plants. Insoluble fiber is wonderful for gastrointestinal health, and even better, soluble fiber can lower your cholesterol and your risk of heart disease if you keep your saturated fat and cholesterol intake low.

If you follow the American Heart Association's recommendations for including fruits, vegetables, and grains in your diet, you should get at least 25 grams of fiber (including both soluble and insoluble) per day. In general, Americans get only half that much. You can get high doses of fiber in kidney beans, pinto beans, potatoes eaten with their skin, green peas, brussels sprouts, broccoli, prunes, apples, oat bran, and brown rice. Breads with whole grains are especially healthful. One study found that three slices of rye bread a day helped reduce the risk of heart disease by 17 percent!

Antioxidants

Antioxidants do exactly what their name implies: They help prevent normal body substances from being oxidized. When LDL (low-density lipoprotein), a cholesterol carrier in the blood, gets oxidized, it is more likely to pile up its cholesterol in the artery wall. Antioxidants, such as vitamins A (beta carotene), C, and E, work by neutralizing the body's unstable molecules (free radicals). Oxidation of these molecules causes cell damage and may contribute to cancer and cataracts, as well as heart disease.

What does this mean to you? Make sure you get plenty of the antioxidant vitamins in your diet. We don't advise spending your money on expensive supplements. Some rich sources of antioxidant vitamins are cantaloupe, guavas, prunes, nectarines, peaches, strawberries, oranges, kiwifruit, mangoes, broccoli, cabbage, asparagus, tomatoes, turnip and other greens, carrots, sweet potatoes, wheat germ, oils and margarines, spinach, melons, winter squash, and nuts, especially hazelnuts and almonds.

Exercise

Exercise goes hand in hand with a healthful diet. Like nutritious foods, it can help lower your risk for heart disease. In fact, inactive people are almost twice as likely as more active people to develop heart disease, according to the U.S. Surgeon General.

The bare minimum of exercise you should get is 30 minutes of moderate activity on most days. If you're sedentary and want to build up, you can start with moderate activities, such as gardening or light housekeeping. If you find that a spare half hour is hard to come by, you can even break your time into 10- or 15-minute segments.

Eating Plans and Shopping

Imagine how it would be if *every* aspect of a meal—the cooking, the eating, and yes, even the planning and shopping for it—were pleasurable. If you're one of the many people who find these last two tasks a particular chore, we can help change your mind. You can make them simpler, faster, and even fun.

A Week of Meals

Sometime each week, have a seat in your favorite chair and make a meal plan for the week. Agreed, this does take some time. However, it also *saves* time and may reduce stress. Thinking ahead keeps you from having to struggle over what to fix for dinner after a difficult day. It also allows you to make one shopping trip instead of three or four (probably at rush hour). Bank on a few family favorites, and take advantage of specials at the supermarket. Try some new flavors to make cooking more exciting. If you want to start meal planning gradually, you can just glance through this cookbook and map out your main courses. Then you can improvise nightly with healthful side dishes, such as whole-grain breads and frozen vegetables, that you have on hand.

If you keep a folder or a notebook for your menu plans, you can refer to the old ones when making a new one. Even allowing for trying different recipes, buying items on sale, and taking advantage of seasonal produce availability, your planning should soon take less time.

The key to a delicious meal is variety. When planning your menus, go for a range of textures and flavors. For example, a crisp salad goes well with a soft casserole, and a spicy or highly flavored entrée is complemented by a simple side dish.

Super Savers

We've come up with four recipe types to turn to when you're in a big hurry to get dinner on the table. They're called New Classics, Planned-

Overs, Shopping Cart recipes, and Express-ipes. Check the descriptions below and the chart on page 14 to find out how they work.

New Classics

These are the standby recipes—the basic main dishes that you can build on or dress up as your mood dictates. The foundation of your repertoire, they are basic recipes for a pound of fish, a pound of chicken breasts, a can of tuna, some lean ground beef, and so on. Some of them also include a variation. You'll probably think of ways to personalize them to match your preferences too. The recipes are simple, use common ingredients, and are so easy to remember that you can practically whip them up in your sleep after a long day. The New Classics icon designates these recipes.

Planned-Overs

When you make soups, stews, or casseroles, you probably already prepare extra for leftovers. Sometimes, though, you get tired of eating the same thing twice in a row. That's why we included Planned-Overs—recipes that use last night's leftovers as a part of tonight's main dish. For example, you could make a lot of Orange-Barbecue Chicken Chunks (page 150) one day, then a couple of days later use the extra for Asian Chicken and Wild Rice Salad (page 84), or transform some of the Tuscan Braised Beef (pages 196–97) into Thai Beef Salad (page 88). Look for the Planned-Overs icon as you leaf through this book.

Shopping Cart Recipes

Shopping Cart recipes are so simple they're almost not recipes at all. Except staples, such as pepper, flour, and acceptable vegetable oil, that you're likely to have on hand, no Shopping Cart recipe calls for more than six common ingredients. That's so they'll be easy enough to remember when you're too rushed to plan ahead or shop ahead and are tempted to get fat-laden, sodium-saturated fast food at the drive-through. Instead, stop at the grocery store and grab the few ingredients you need for your favorite Shopping Cart entrée. Little if any cooking is needed, so you'll be in and out of the kitchen in almost no time. For example, you can easily pick up in one grocery store all the ingredients you need for Italian Bean and Tuna Salad (page 81). When you get home, toss everything into a bowl, and presto! Dinner is ready. Look for the Shopping Cart icon on these main-dish recipes.

Express-ipes

The quickest of the quick, the easiest of the easy, these entrées are ready in 25 minutes or less. That's 25 minutes for *all* the preparation and *all* the cooking, if there is any. Many are ready in much less time. For example, Pizza Soup (page 60) clocks in at a total time of only 10 minutes, start to finish, and Honey Mustard Salmon (page117) takes only 11. Look for the Express-ipes icon ▨ when you want a real time-saver. They're faster—and cheaper—than fast food.

Look for this . . .	When you want . . .	So you can . . .
	a New Classics recipe	Make a quick main dish from what's on hand. Many of these offer at least one variation to satisfy your hunger for whatever flavor you crave.
	a Planned-Overs recipe	Use leftovers to create a totally different dish. This is our twofer concept.
	a Shopping Cart recipe	Buy six or fewer items at the grocery store and whip up an entrée pronto. Use this for a day when it's time for dinner and you have nothing planned.
	an Express-ipe	Have your entrée ready—start to finish—in 25 minutes or less.

Another helpful type of recipe to include in your weekly plan is the All-in-One. It combines meat or a meat substitute, at least one vegetable, and a carbohydrate of some sort—and it usually requires only one pot or pan.

Serve these recipes with simple sides, such as whole-wheat rolls and fresh fruit, or make salad or dessert while the dish is cooking. Look for the All-in-One icon ❶ to find these recipes.

Shopping Savvy

If you dislike grocery shopping, it may be that you forget to set yourself up for success. Perhaps you shop when you're hungry, when the store is crowded, or when you don't have a list.

To avoid these pitfalls, the first step is to make a list that's organized according to the store layout. You can even ask the manager for a map of the store and make multiple copies. Using a clean copy for each weekly trip, write down the items you need on the aisles where you'll find them. Use the maps as a time-saver when you need just a few nonstandard items too. It's a lot faster to check the map than to go up and down the aisles until you happen upon the caramel topping.

An alternative is to list on your computer the foods you buy most often. List them in the order they're in at the store, leaving space for additions. Print out a copy each week and circle the items you need. The printed list also serves as a reminder. Do you need carrots this week? orange juice? vegetable oil spray? If you keep your fridge, freezer, and pantry well stocked with the basics, perhaps by keeping a copy of that list or a pad of paper and a pencil handy in the kitchen, you'll be less likely to run out of a needed ingredient in the middle of preparing a dish. This certainly reduces frustration and cuts down on frantic trips to the supermarket.

A good time to shop is about 8 P.M., after most shoppers are already home. Early morning is another quick time. During Sunday afternoon football may be a good time in your neighborhood. If you go at 5 P.M., when most people get off work, you'll encounter lines. You're also more likely to be hungry and therefore tempted by fatty, empty-calorie treats you don't need.

Consider buying food in the form you'll use—shredded cheese, chopped vegetables, boned and skinned chicken breasts. Also, the salad bars at large supermarkets can be a real time-saver. Among many other possibilities, you're likely to find already-washed, torn spinach, romaine, and leaf lettuce; thinly sliced radishes and celery; shredded carrots; and chopped onion. Prepared items may cost more than in their original, whole form, but they'll save you time and perhaps cut down on waste. You buy only what you need, so there are no tough outer leaves or heavy stems to toss out, and there's no half bunch of celery to discard after it shrivels up.

With easy ingredients for easy meals so readily available, you'll be less tempted to give up on cooking and order takeout.

What to Look For

Here are some guidelines to help you skirt the fat-laden goodies and fill your cart with heart-healthy treats.

Meat

Look at the label when buying meat. Cuts called Prime have the most fat, those that say Select have the least, and Choice meats are in between. Good beef choices are flank steak, sirloin, sirloin tip, tenderloin, round steak, and extra lean ground beef (we used ground beef with 10 percent fat in our nutrient analyses). The best choices in pork include tenderloin, loin chops, Canadian bacon, and center-cut ham. In lamb, you want the meat to be finely grained and reddish pink. The leanest cuts are sirloin chop, center roast, center slice, and shank. Veal's leanest cuts are leg cutlet, arm steak, sirloin steak, rib chop, loin chop, and top round.

Poultry

White meat has less fat than dark, and turkey has less than chicken. Cornish hens are another good choice. Whatever kind of poultry you choose, it's really important that you don't eat the skin, where most of the fat and calories are.

Seafood

Some of the leanest fish are cod, haddock, halibut, flounder, sole, red snapper, and orange roughy. Canned tuna is easy to use; just look for tuna packed in distilled or spring water. Fatty fish may be slightly more caloric, but their omega-3 fatty acids may reduce your risk of heart disease. (See "Basics of a Healthful Diet," pages 5–11.) Some fish high in omega-3 fatty acids are Atlantic and coho salmon, albacore tuna, mackerel, and lake and brook trout. Most shellfish are very low in fat. Shrimp and crawfish are higher in cholesterol than most other seafood but are lower in fat than most meats and poultry.

Dairy

As you would guess, fat-free milk is the best kind to buy. If an old favorite recipe calls for light cream, you can simply substitute fat-free evaporated milk. It's perfect in sauces. Both nonfat and light sour cream work well in hot and cold recipes. Among cheeses, it's best to leave the worst fat offenders—Brie, Camembert, and cheese spreads—in the dairy case, except occasionally. Cheeses naturally low in fat are part-skim mozzarella, farmer, part-skim ricotta, and Parmesan. For most other cheeses (including favorites such as Cheddar and Monterey Jack), look for fat-free and reduced-fat versions. When shopping for cottage or cream cheese, look for the ones that are fat free or low fat. If you're watching your sodium intake, remember that nonfat cheeses are generally higher in that department. Finally, if dessert is on your mind, delicious substitutes for ice cream are ice milk, nonfat or low-fat ice cream or frozen yogurt, sherbet, and fruit ices.

Eggs

As we've already mentioned, egg yolks are high in cholesterol. Just one contains about 213 milligrams—two-thirds of your full daily allowance. You may want to pick up a carton of egg substitute.

Vegetables and Fruits

Most fruits and vegetables have little or no fat, and they're low in sodium and high in fiber and vitamins. The exceptions are coconuts, which are high in saturated fat, and avocados, which are high in mono-unsaturated fat. Eat these in moderation.

As far as packaged vegetables go, stir-fry mixes in the frozen food or the produce section are great for quick side dishes. Look carefully at the nutrient information for the packets of sauce that sometimes come with the mixes. If the sauce is high in sodium, you may want to make your own instead. Presliced mushrooms and prewashed and bagged salad greens and coleslaw mixtures will save you lots of prep time. Lettuces sold in bulk, however, need to be cleaned.

Frozen fruit is wonderful for smoothies and desserts. When possible, use the kind without added sugar. If you have a choice, select fruit canned in water or its own juice rather than in syrup.

An incredible number of exotic fruits and vegetables that most of us hadn't even heard of just a few years ago are now widely available. When you don't have to make a mad dash through the supermarket, take a look at what's new. You may be able to entice the kids—or yourself—to try something different.

Breads and Cereals

Since breads and cereals comprise the bulk of the Healthy Heart Food Pyramid way of eating, you'll want to stock up on them. Check the labels to help find bread products that don't contain egg yolks. Try to choose whole-grain breads, since they contain more nutrients and fiber. "Wheat" bread is not whole-wheat bread. Look for labels that say "100% whole wheat" or that list whole-wheat flour as one of the first few ingredients.

Flashy cereal packaging can be tempting, but read the labels. Look for cereals that have 3 or fewer grams of fat per ounce and are a good source of fiber.

If you're cooking in a hurry, you can always buy instant rice. Naturally fast cooking pastas and grains, including couscous and bulgur, are flavorful alternatives. Bags of dried beans and lentils are good to have around to replace meat in stews and casseroles, or use no-salt-added canned beans to conserve time. When those aren't available, rinse regular canned beans to get rid of extra sodium. In our recipes, we call for rinsing even no-salt-added canned beans because lots of people prefer the flavor that way. You can skip this step if you wish.

Snacks

The best snacks of all are fruits and veggies. If you have to have a chip fix, choose baked chips. Unsalted seeds and nuts are good for you, but they're high in total fat and calories. Eat them in moderation.

Miscellaneous

Quick and easy cooks often stock the cupboard with canned goods. Many canned items are loaded with sodium, so watch labels carefully. You may notice that some of our recipes first call for no-salt-added canned goods and then call for salt. The simple reason is that the end result is far less sodium than you'd have from using the regular canned product and no salt.

Other high-sodium foods to limit are salsa; soy sauce; steak sauce; spaghetti, pasta, and marinara sauces; flour tortillas; ketchup; chili sauce; pickles; and relishes. Look at the labels to find the ones with the lowest sodium. It's worth the search—similar products can vary greatly.

You'll find that our recipes never call for meat tenderizer or cooking wine. Both are just too high in sodium to use.

Fresh herbs, citrus juices, and garlic are more flavorful than dried herbs, bottled juices, and dehydrated or bottled garlic, but they take a little longer to prepare. Since this cookbook has "quick" and "easy" in its subtitle, we almost always list the faster varieties first.

Nutrition Labels

No matter how hurried your shopping may be, always try to pause to read the labels. All U.S.–made packaged foods have them, and they're jam-packed with useful information that can make regulating your fat, sugar, cholesterol, sodium, and vitamin intake a breeze. The U.S. government monitors food labeling, so serving sizes are uniform across all brands.

Nutrition Facts

Serving Size ½ cup (114g)
Servings Per Container 4

Amount Per Serving

Calories 90   Calories from Fat 30

	% Daily Value*
Total Fat 3g	**5%**
Saturated Fat 0g	**0%**
Cholesterol 0mg	**0%**
Sodium 300mg	**13%**
Total Carbohydrate 13g	**4%**
Dietary Fiber 3g	**12%**
Sugars 3g	
Protein 3g	

Vitamin A	80%	•	Vitamin C	60%
Calcium	4%	•	Iron	4%

*Percent Daily Values are based on a 2,000 calorie diet. Your daily values may be higher or lower depending on your calorie needs:

	Calories	2,000	2,500
Total Fat	Less than	65g	80g
	Less than	20g	25g
Cholesterol	Less than	300mg	300mg
Sodium	Less than	2,400mg	2,400mg
Total Carbohydrate		300g	375g
		25g	30g

Calories per gram:
Fat 9   •   Carbohydrate 4   •   Protein 4

The first stop on your label scan should be the ingredients list. Contents are listed according to weight; the largest amount comes first and the smallest, last. Watch for fats, sodium, or sugars too high on the list. Fat sources to look out for include cocoa butter, coconut, coconut oil, palm oil, and palm kernel oil. Some sources of "hidden salt" are soy sauce and baking soda. Others are substances with the word "sodium" in their name. Two examples are monosodium glutamate, or MSG, and sodium bicarbonate. Any word ending with "-ose," such as "lactose" or "sucrose," indicates a sugar in disguise.

Here's the other important information you'll find on the label:

Serving size: Serving sizes across all similar foods are consistent. That lets you comparison shop, looking for the most heart-healthy choices. If you double a serving, remember to double everything else on the label too.

Calories and calories from fat: This is a quick count of the calories in the serving as a whole and of those that come specifically from fat.

Daily values for nutrients: The government uses a 2,000-calorie diet to determine the limits on nutrients you should eat every day. The section of the label for percentage of daily values shows how well a product stacks up. It lists nutrients, followed by the daily percentage a serving of this food provides. For example, if a nutrient is followed by "100%," you're getting all you need for the day. If it's one of the nutrients with a minimum limit and the value is less than 100%, you'll need to look to other foods to make up the difference. The nutrients listed are total fat, saturated fat, cholesterol, sodium, total carbohydrate, dietary fiber, and vitamins A and C, as well as calcium and iron. Others, such as sugars and mono- and polyunsaturated fats, sometimes are listed.

Key Words on Food Labels and What They Mean

The government regulates the claims that food manufacturers make. Following are a few terms you'll often see on labels.

Key words	What they mean
Fat-free	Less than 0.5 gram of fat per serving
Low-fat	3 grams of fat or less per serving
Lean	Less than 10 grams of fat, 4.5 grams of saturated fat, and 95 milligrams of cholesterol per serving

EATING PLANS AND SHOPPING

Light (lite)	One-third fewer calories or no more than half the fat of the higher-calorie, higher-fat version; or no more than half the sodium of the higher-sodium version
Cholesterol-free	Less than 2 milligrams of cholesterol and 2 grams or less of saturated fat per serving

Labeling Regulations for Health Claims

Federal regulations also set specific standards for health claims manufacturers may include on food labels.

To make claims about . . .	The food must be . . .
Heart disease and fats and cholesterol	Low in fat, saturated fat, and cholesterol
Blood pressure and sodium	Low in sodium
Heart disease and fruits, vegetables, and grain products that contain fiber	Low in fat, saturated fat, and cholesterol and contain at least 0.6 gram soluble fiber, without fortification, per serving

Food Certification Program

You'll notice that some food labels sport a heart with a check mark through it.

This means that the food meets the American Heart Association criteria for saturated fat and cholesterol levels for healthy people over age two. When you see this symbol, you know you're buying a heart-smart product.

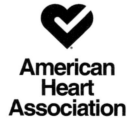

American Heart Association

Meets American Heart Association food criteria for saturated fat and cholesterol for healthy people over age 2.

Getting Organized

Take a good look at your kitchen. Is it a place you love to be in? a place full of accessible tools you enjoy both looking at and using? a place where everything *has* a place? If not, it's time to make it that way. An organized kitchen is so much more peaceful and so much less stressful than a disorderly kitchen that you'll be glad you made the effort.

Let's start with the clutter. Take a deep breath and clear it away. Mail and homework that have a way of creeping onto a countertop also have a way of making meal preparation hectic. Get rid of any utensils you no longer use. Face it—if you have a gizmo you haven't picked up in two years, you'll probably never use it again. If you put dividers in your utensil drawers, you'll be able to reach for that slotted spoon or pair of tongs without getting lost in a tangle of metal. Try hanging your most-used skillets and saucepans on a pegboard or hooks for the same reason. It's all part of your goal: an easy stage for an easy meal.

When you stand at your stove and countertop, is everything you need within quick reach? Cooking will go more smoothly if the necessities are nearby—potholders hanging near the stove and the microwave, and knives organized on a magnetic rack or in a block near the cutting area. If you need more space, try putting drawers or turntables in the lower cabinets.

Prepping Made Easy

Now that you've organized your kitchen, let's look at the way you start a meal.

The first step is reading the recipes thoroughly—at least once. Next, it helps to devise a timing strategy if you're cooking more than one dish. Most cooks agree that you should pull out all the necessary ingredients and line them up on the counter. The French call this *mise en place* ("everything in its place"), and it helps curb mid-preparation panic when you suddenly realize you have no baking powder for the cake you've already begun. It also helps keep you from forgetting to use an ingredient. Go one more step and assemble the utensils you'll need too. That will save steps and, consequently, time.

Tools of the Trade

Every kitchen (and every cook!) is different, but here are the tools of the trade most well-prepped, speedy chefs consider essential.

- Several high-quality knives and a knife sharpener.
- A large skillet with a tight-fitting lid.
- A pan you can use both on the stovetop and in the oven.
- A few nonstick pots and pans. You need little or no oil with these, and they're easier to clean.
- A Dutch oven.
- Two dishwasher-safe chopping boards.
- An electric slow cooker. It may not be fast, but it sure is easy. And when you come home from work, your house will be full of delicious smells!
- A nest of mixing bowls.
- A whisk, a big spoon, a slotted spoon, kitchen scissors, tongs, and spatulas.
- Clearly marked measuring spoons and measuring cups.

Freezer Basics

Your freezer should be more than a holding cell for leftovers. You can also use it to store the building blocks for many recipes, preserved for freshness and always on hand. Try to designate a specific area of the freezer for these basic items. Whether you have only a refrigerator freezer or a separate unit as well, knowing just where to reach for an item instead of rooting around for it will be a tremendous time-saver. It won't take any more space to be organized than to be a frazzled cook. You might even want to buy a freezerproof plastic container to hold your freezer staples. Here are some foods to consider always keeping on hand.

Cubes of low-sodium chicken, beef, and vegetable broth are almost essential for quick, healthful cooks. Measure broth by the tablespoonful into the compartments of an ice cube tray, freeze, and then pop out the cubes. Keep them frozen in airtight freezer bags. Whenever you need to sauté, toss a cube into the pan (no need to thaw first). It's much more healthful than using oil.

Those trays can also be used for freezing tablespoonfuls of lemon, lime, and orange juice. To get more juice, roll the fruit on the counter, pressing gently, before squeezing.

Since so many recipes require tomato paste, yet you rarely use a whole can, why not freeze it by the tablespoonful too? Freeze the tomato paste dollops on a cookie sheet, then store them in an airtight plastic freezer bag.

Chicken breasts are a must. If you go ahead and remove the skin and all the visible fat now, you'll be so glad you did when prep time rolls around and you're in a big hurry. Boneless breasts can be pounded and stacked in layers, separated by sheets of wax paper so it's easy to remove as many or as few as you wish from the freezer.

Grated cheese keeps well in the freezer. (Frozen blocks of cheese tend to crumble when thawed and, therefore, can be difficult to slice.) Store grated cheese in airtight plastic freezer bags, and you'll save yourself some labor at mealtime. It's cheaper to buy blocks of cheese and grate your own than to buy grated cheese.

Onions and bell peppers of various colors are great to have around. Chop extra when you have a minute or when they're on sale, then store them in the freezer. If you prefer, buy frozen chopped onions or frozen chopped or sliced peppers.

Even cooked pasta freezes easily. Toss it with a tiny bit of oil to keep it from sticking. When you want to eat the pasta, just drop it into boiling water for about two minutes. For many varieties, this way is much faster than starting from scratch!

Buy berries in season, when they're most flavorful and least expensive. To freeze berries, place them, separated, on a baking sheet. When they're frozen, toss them into airtight plastic freezer bags. The berries will be terrific in smoothies, desserts, breads, and even soups.

Cooking for a Healthy Heart

Since the way you prepare a dish is as important as the ingredients you put into it, you won't find recipes for deep-fried anything in this cookbook. Here's a guide to many wonderful cooking methods that are much more healthful for your heart and still pleasing to your palate.

- *Broiling:* Broiling cooks food quickly at a very high heat and lets the fat drip away. Most seafood and meat, sliced thin, will broil in 5 to 10 minutes. Broiling also is a great method for getting tender, delicious vegetables. Healthful alternatives to butter for basting include low-sodium broth, fruit juice, flavored vinegar, and wine.
- *Grilling:* When you cook on a grill, the fat can easily drip away while the smoke subtly imparts flavor to the food. The same liquids used in basting while broiling are appropriate in grilling.
- *Sautéing:* If you are using a nonstick pan, heat it, then add a small amount of low-sodium broth, juice, wine, or acceptable oil or margarine, and quickly sauté the food without crowding. With a regular pan, heat it, move it away from the heat, and then lightly spray it with vegetable oil spray (the spray is flammable). Add liquid and sauté the food.
- *Stir-frying:* Stir-frying is similar to sautéing in that both are quick methods of cooking that require little liquid. In both methods, the food shouldn't be crowded in the pan. Stir-frying uses higher heat and almost constant stirring. A small amount of oil is almost always used. Stir-frying works well with most vegetables and most types of meat, poultry, and seafood.
- *Baking:* Good for poultry and fish, baking is simple and straightforward. Put your food in a dish, put the dish in the oven, and go about your business. Many recipes call for covering the dish and adding liquid to keep the food from becoming dry.
- *Braising:* Braising is a slow-cooking method that tenderizes meat and lets the fat cook out. It's also good for vegetables. First,

brown the food. Then cook it, tightly covered, in a little liquid for a long time over low heat. If you braise your meat dish a day ahead and then chill it, the fat will rise to the top and congeal for easy removal.

■ *Steaming:* Steaming is an excellent way to cook veggies and fish while preserving the food's flavor, as well as its vitamins and minerals. A steamer basket or a rack, a small amount of boiling or simmering water, and a pan with a tight-fitting lid do the trick. The food goes in the basket or on the rack over the water. The bottom of the basket or the rack shouldn't touch the water. Cover the pan and cook for a few minutes, and your food will be perfectly steamed.

■ *Poaching:* Poaching is a great way to cook chicken or fish, because the meat stays moist as it's gently simmered in a liquid. Bring low-sodium stock, wine, or fruit juice to a bubble over low heat, add your meat, and voilà! Your meal will be infused with real flavor.

■ *Microwave cooking:* The microwave is both fast and easy for so many kinds of food. When you keep the food covered as it cooks, it produces its own moisture, so you don't have to add any fats or oils.

About These Recipes

With an eye on speed and ease, we've made sure that the preparation time for each recipe is no more than 20 minutes from the moment you set foot in the kitchen. Bear in mind, though, that every cook works at a different speed and that you'll probably get faster after you've made a dish a time or two. The lengths of prep time are based on several assumptions. For one thing, we assume that your kitchen is pretty well organized (see "Getting Organized," pages 22–24) and that you have a food processor or a blender. We also imagine that quick cooks buy certain convenience foods, such as grated cheese and frozen chopped onions. If these guesses aren't true in your case, you'll need to add a bit of time to our numbers.

Many recipes in this cookbook will be table-ready within a half hour after you begin. Others, of course, take more time to cook or need longer chilling or baking time. Prep time and cooking time are given separately for each recipe. If applicable, so are chilling, freezing, standing, and cooling times.

Please keep in mind that the sum may be more than its parts. Whenever possible, we'll direct you to prep one part of a dish while another part cooks. That's why you can't necessarily add up all the listed times and assume that the total is how long you'll be cooking.

Each recipe will walk you through exactly what you need to do. Although many cooks advise prepping all ingredients first, we may, for example, have you chop the mushrooms up front, then slice the carrots as the mushrooms sauté. We think that minimizes downtime.

Are you ever annoyed when a recipe says you'll need, for example, 6 cups of torn fresh spinach? Do you take a chance and eyeball that amount at the grocery store, or do you search through your cookbooks in hope of finding an equivalents list that will tell you how many ounces of spinach to buy? To help you shop and prep, we put amounts in parentheses after certain ingredients. Those numbers show you how much to buy—and later take out of the fridge, freezer, or pantry—to get the amount you need. We'll say "6 cups torn spinach (about 8 ounces)" in the ingredients list. You might see "2 cups sliced carrots (2 large)" in the ingredients list even though 1½ large carrots equal 2 cups. That's because you would need to have two carrots, not one, on hand. If you'll need only one or less than one of an ingredient, we don't give the equivalent. Please note that the equivalents are based on averages.

We also list amounts for both eggs and egg substitute if a recipe yields ¼ egg or less per serving. If it yields more, we list only the substitute amount.

Nutrient Analysis

Each recipe has been analyzed for calories, protein, carbohydrates, cholesterol, total fat, saturated fat, polyunsaturated fat, monounsaturated fat, fiber, and sodium. You can use this analysis to quickly determine how well the dish will fit into your overall eating plan and needs.

Everyone tends to calculate analyses like these slightly differently; here's how we did ours.

- Each analysis is based on a single serving, unless we indicate otherwise.
- We didn't include garnishes or optional ingredients in the nutrient analysis unless they would significantly change the amount of one or more nutrients. In those few instances, you'll find an analysis for the dish with the extra ingredients as well as without them.
- The beautiful photographs in this book may be garnished to enhance the looks of the dish. Those garnishes also aren't included. We highly recommend the use of garnishes for everyday as well as company meals—even quick meals; making the effort to make your dish more appealing to the eye will help you savor the moment. Just remember that if you eat it, you need to count it. That's especially true if the garnish would bump up the numbers for saturated fat, cholesterol, or sodium.
- When we provided a range with our ingredients (a 2½- to 3-pound chicken, for example), we analyzed the average.
- When we list ingredient options (½ cup fat-free or low-fat yogurt, for instance), we used the *first* for the nutrient analysis.
- When a recipe calls for acceptable margarine, we used corn oil margarine for the analysis. (Remember to choose a margarine that lists liquid vegetable oil as the first ingredient.)
- When a recipe calls for acceptable vegetable oil, we used corn oil. Other acceptable vegetable oils include canola, olive, safflower, sesame, soybean, and sunflower. If you prefer one of them,

feel free to substitute it. For an occasional change of flavor when you need an oil that doesn't smoke until it's *really* hot, you can use peanut oil.

■ The values for saturated, monounsaturated, and polyunsaturated fats may not add up precisely to the amount listed for total fat in the recipe. That's because we rounded to whole numbers and because total fat includes other fatty substances and glycerol as well.

■ If a nutrient analysis shows a dash instead of a number for polyunsaturated or monounsaturated fat, this means those values weren't available for at least one ingredient in the recipe.

■ For our reduced-fat cheese analysis, we figured in cheese with 3 or fewer grams of fat per serving. If you'd like to cut down even further, choose fat-free cheese, which has less than 0.5 gram of fat per serving.

■ Meat statistics were based on cooked lean meat with all visible fat removed. Lean ground beef was 90 percent fat free.

■ Analyses of recipes with meat marinades include only the amount absorbed by the meat, based on United States Department of Agriculture (USDA) data on absorption. If the marinade is boiled and then used for basting or in a sauce, we include the full amount of all the ingredients.

■ Although data are available to show how much sodium is lost when foods such as canned green beans and cottage cheese are rinsed (and we use those data in our nutrient analyses), they aren't available for foods such as olives, capers, feta cheese, and bottled roasted red bell peppers. We suggest rinsing those foods, however, because we feel that will get rid of some sodium.
If you do so, you can assume that the sodium level in recipes containing these salty foods is a little lower than the nutrient analyses indicate.

■ As we discuss in "Key Words on Food Labels and What They Mean" (pages 19–20), foods can't be called low sodium ("light" or "lite"), for example, unless they meet certain government criteria. That's why you probably won't find salsa, spaghetti sauce, pizza sauce, or nonfat flour tortillas with labels saying they're low sodium or satay sauce labeled "low fat." When you're shopping for these products, however, be sure to compare label information and choose the products that are lowest in fat, saturated fat, cholesterol, and sodium. That's what we did in our analyses.

■ Unless specified otherwise, all measurements are level.

- We use the abbreviations for "gram" (g) and for "milligram" (mg).
- You still can count on the analyses when you make substitutions that don't affect a recipe's basic nutritional profile. For example, you can substitute fresh lemon juice for reconstituted or try tarragon vinegar instead of white wine vinegar.

Because the products calculated in the nutrient analyses may not be exactly the same as those you used, you'll need to consider all analyses as approximate. For instance, the analysis may be based on Brand X but you may have used Brand Y. Even though their labels say both are low-fat raspberry vinaigrette, the products are unlikely to have exactly the same values for each nutrient we list in the nutrient analysis.

Cook's Tips

Whether you're a novice or a seasoned cook, we think there's always something new to learn. That's why you'll find Cook's Tips with many of our recipes.

Some tips are recipe-specific; that is, they apply only to the recipe with which they appear. Such tips might divulge ways to prepare the recipes more easily or give storage tips.

Most of the tips are more general, so you can use what you learn in a variety of recipes. Among other things, these tips tell ways to simplify procedures, where to find and how to use unusual ingredients, and what to do with leftovers.

Time-Savers

You might wonder why a quick and easy cookbook needs timesaving tips. We've included a handful of these to explain, for example, why we suggest doing one step before another or how the use of alternative ingredients can sometimes speed up a process.

Now you know some of the tricks of the trade we used to put this book together. It's your turn! Use these recipes to create wonderful meals you, your family, and your friends will enjoy.

Top Tips of Our Super Chefs

Who better knows how to save time in the kitchen than the people who work there? That's why we asked our team of recipe developers for their most valued timesaving tips—the tricks they turn to again and again when they need to shave a few minutes off meal preparation and cleanup. Here's what they said:

- Use wide skillets and higher temperatures to speed up a sauté. A wide skillet helps any liquid evaporate, so the food cooks more quickly. Covering the skillet also speeds up the process.
- Sharpen your knives regularly to make chopping quick and easy. You're actually more likely to cut yourself with a dull knife than with a sharp one.
- If you have a lot of chopping to do, use a food processor. If you need to chop only a small amount, use a mini processor or a sharp knife to save on cleanup time.
- Before you start cooking, fill the sink with hot, soapy water. This way, you can drop bowls and utensils in as you go. They'll be easy to clean if you need them again as you cook.
- Set a single sheet of wax paper curved side down on your work surface. It makes a handy place to set down messy spoons and spatulas. You can then just throw away one piece of wax paper, rather than having to scrub a whole counter. Lightly wiping the counter with a moist paper towel helps keep the wax paper in place.
- Another sheet of wax paper is handy if you're grating cheese or lemon peel. Aim for the measuring cup or spoon as you grate; then spoon the "misses" from the wax paper into the implement. This method also works well when you're measuring flour and confectioners' sugar.
- A damp paper towel under your cutting board helps keep the board in place.

- To bring water to a boil faster, start with hot tap water and cover the pot. If you're using a lot of water, divide it between two pots until it starts boiling.
- Store your utensils near where you're most likely to use them. For instance, it's handy to keep your long-handled spoons, whisks, and soup ladle near the stove.
- Except when baking foods such as cakes and yeast breads, for which precision is the key to success, you hardly ever need to obsess about ingredients. If a recipe says to slice carrots but you have some already chopped, use them. If it calls for oregano and you have basil, chances are overwhelmingly in your favor that the results will be fine. It isn't worth taking the time to rush to the store during peak shopping times to get the "right" ingredient.
- You can roast vegetables, such as bell peppers and onions, while you roast or bake other things. If you won't need the veggies soon, freeze them for later use.
- Another way to make double use of your time is to boil noodles for tomorrow's pasta salad while cooking or cleaning up for today.
- Remove the visible fat from boneless, skinless chicken breasts before freezing the chicken.
- Measure dry ingredients before wet ones so you can reuse measuring spoons and cups without having to wash them between steps.
- Keep high-intensity, flavorful ingredients on hand. It takes no time to throw in a tablespoon of mint, pine nuts, currants, or olives, any of which can make a simple dish outstanding.
- Put your herbs and spices in alphabetical order. This works especially well if you have lots of them and/or you can't see all of them at a glance. You'll save time by not having to search for the right jar.
- Take full advantage of all the services the butcher may offer. He or she will usually chop or prepare any meat to your specifications, free of charge. You can even call ahead with your request. If, for example, a dish calls for 12 ounces of steak, thinly sliced, ask for that specifically. Then all you have to do when you get home is slide the meat out of the package and trim the visible fat.
- The same goes for seafood. If you call ahead, a butcher will usually peel your shrimp for you. Check to see whether there will be a charge for this service.

- Make use of supermarket salad bars. The produce is fresh, clean, and already sliced, chopped, or torn. Some produce department personnel will even take phone orders for prepping fruits and vegetables for you.
- Put your frozen vegetables in a colander under cold running water (not hot, which would cook them slightly) for 15 to 20 seconds. This refreshes them and makes them cook faster.
- Keep emergency meals on hand for those nights when you're just too tired to cook. Veggie burgers are a good option, as are left-over casseroles, soups, and stews.
- Make time for cooking rather than finding time. If you cook meals that you enjoy, using ingredients you love, you won't mind spending a few extra minutes in the kitchen.

You and your family are about to have the pleasure of eating a variety of attractive, wholesome foods while nourishing your bodies for health and daily activities. Enjoy!

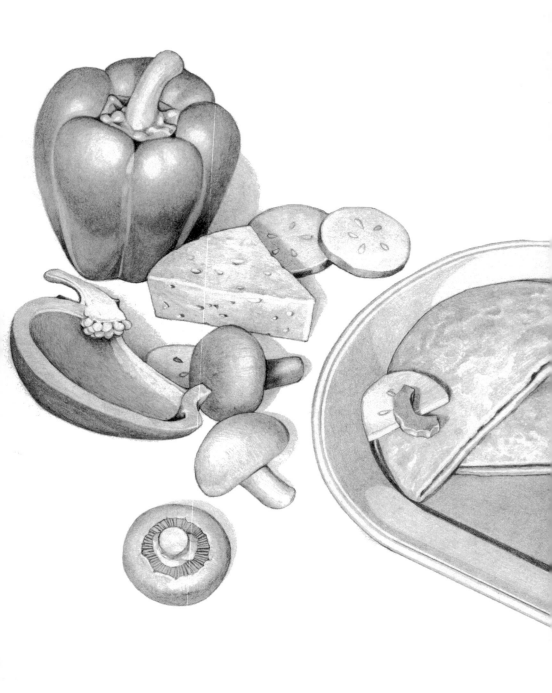

Appetizers, Snacks, and Beverages

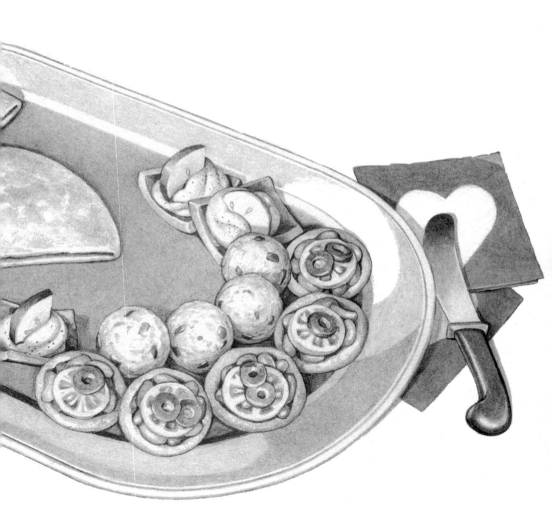

■ ■ ■

Dill and Sour Cream Dip

Mexican Bean Dip

Mini Vegetable Cheese Balls

Cheese-Filled Bell Pepper Boats

Roasted Vegetable Spread

Italian Quiche in Phyllo Shells

Turkey Potstickers

Stacked Mushroom Nachos

Morning Energy Drink

 Morning Energy "Soup"

Pineapple Shakes

 Orange Shakes

Strawberry Mint Spritzer

 Strawberry Mint Smoothie

■ ■ ■

Dill and Sour Cream Dip

The subtle, fresh taste of dill is at its best when teamed with cucumbers. Cut some into spears, rounds, or wedges and try them with this super-simple dip.

¾ cup nonfat or light sour cream

1 tablespoon plus 1½ teaspoons snipped fresh dillweed or 1½ teaspoons dried, crumbled

1 tablespoon lemon juice

1 tablespoon extra-virgin olive oil

¼ teaspoon salt

In a small bowl, whisk together all ingredients.
Serve or cover and refrigerate until serving time.

(PER SERVING)

Calories 42

Protein 1 g

Carbohydrates 5 g

Cholesterol 3 mg

Total Fat 2 g

  Saturated 0 g

   Polyunsaturated 0 g

   Monounsaturated 1 g

Fiber 0 g

Sodium 117 mg

Mexican Bean Dip

- Serves 6; ¼ cup per serving
- Preparation time: 10 minutes

You can enjoy this protein- and fiber-packed, easy-to-prepare dip on salt-free baked tortilla chips for a quick appetizer or in Vegetarian Taco Salad (page 89) as an entrée.

16-ounce can no-salt-added black beans, rinsed and drained (about 1¼ cups)

½ cup frozen chopped green bell pepper or 1 small green bell pepper, coarsely chopped

¼ cup coarsely chopped fresh cilantro or parsley (optional)

2 tablespoons salsa

2 tablespoons lime juice (1 to 2 medium limes)

1 teaspoon bottled minced garlic or 2 medium cloves garlic, coarsely chopped

1 teaspoon chili powder

½ teaspoon ground cumin

In a food processor or blender, process all ingredients for 45 seconds, or until fairly smooth.

Serve or cover and refrigerate until serving time.

COOK'S TIP ON CANNED BEANS

To give canned beans a clean taste, pour them into a colander and rinse with cool running water until all the bubbles have disappeared. If salt was added to the beans during processing, rinsing will remove a lot of the sodium.

(PER SERVING)

Calories 77

Protein 5 g

Carbohydrates 14 g

Cholesterol 0 mg

Total Fat 1 g

Saturated 0 g

Polyunsaturated 0 g

Monounsaturated 0 g

Fiber 3 g

Sodium 22 mg

Mini Vegetable Cheese Balls

Serves 6; 2 cheese balls per serving ■
Preparation time: 20 minutes ■

Don't let the small size of these cheese balls fool you. They're loaded with flavor and crunch! They're delicious alone, or surround them with toasted pita wedges.

½ cup bell pepper (any color), diced or minced

1 rib celery, diced or minced (about ½ cup)

2 green onions, thinly sliced (about ¼ cup)

2 ounces fat-free cream cheese, softened (¼ cup)

2 tablespoons goat cheese

¼ teaspoon garlic powder

½ cup finely snipped fresh parsley

In a medium bowl, stir together all ingredients except parsley.

Put parsley on a plate. Using a round tablespoon measure, scoop up 1 scant tablespoon cheese mixture. Roll into a ball. Roll ball in parsley, turning to coat. Shake off excess parsley. Repeat with remaining cheese mixture.

Serve or cover and refrigerate until serving time.

Cook's Tip

You can do most of the cheese ball preparation up to 24 hours in advance. Combine the ingredients as directed, then roll the mixture into balls. Cover and refrigerate. Roll the balls in parsley up to 8 hours before serving.

Time-Saver

To save time, make a tasty cheese spread instead of balls. Transfer the cheese mixture to a serving dish, sprinkle with ¼ cup finely snipped parsley, and serve with low-sodium crackers.

(PER SERVING)

Calories 31
Protein 3 g
Carbohydrates 2 g
Cholesterol 4 mg
Total Fat 1 g
  Saturated 1 g
  Polyunsaturated 0 g
  Monounsaturated 0 g
Fiber 1 g
Sodium 96 mg

Cheese-Filled Bell Pepper Boats

- Serves 8; 3 pieces per serving
- Preparation time: 15 minutes

When the colorful allure of the many bell pepper varieties draws you in at the super-market's produce section, try this recipe for an unusual vegetable tray. The cream cheese mixture is also wonderful on celery, on unpeeled cucumber rounds, or in hollowed-out cherry tomato halves.

½ cup fat-free cream cheese, softened (4 ounces)

2 tablespoons shredded or grated Parmesan cheese

1 teaspoon lime juice

1-inch crosswise slice English cucumber

2 medium bell peppers (any colors)

½ teaspoon chili powder

In a small bowl, stir together cream cheese, Parmesan, and lime juice. Spoon mixture into a piping bag fitted with a wide star or round tip.

Thinly slice cucumber crosswise into 12 pieces, then cut each piece in half; set aside.

Cut bell peppers in half, stem end to root end; remove stems, ribs, and seeds. Cut each half into six pieces. Lay pieces skin side down on a serving platter.

Pipe about 1 teaspoon cream cheese mixture onto each square. Sprinkle with chili powder. Stand a cucumber piece in cream cheese mixture on each square.

VARIATION

Substitute small, feathery pieces of fresh dillweed for the chili powder and cucumber.

COOK'S TIP ON DISPOSABLE PIPING, OR PASTRY, BAGS

For easy cleanup, use disposable plastic piping bags or a sturdy sterile plastic bag with a bottom corner snipped off.

(PER SERVING)

Calories 27

Protein 3 g

Carbohydrates 2 g

Cholesterol 4 mg

Total Fat 0 g

　Saturated 0 g

　Polyunsaturated 0 g

　Monounsaturated 0 g

Fiber 0 g

Sodium 126 mg

Roasted Vegetable Spread

Serves 8; 2 tablespoons per serving ■
Preparation time: 15 minutes ■
Cooking time: 20 to 25 minutes ■

*With their slightly caramelized flavor, roasted vegetables make a wonderful spread.
Serve with pieces of toasted pita rounds or baked tortilla chips.*

Olive oil spray

1 medium zucchini, cut in half lengthwise

1 medium crookneck squash, cut in half lengthwise

1 medium carrot, cut into ¼-inch slices

1 medium onion, quartered

2 ounces asparagus, bottom 1 inch trimmed

2 medium Italian plum tomatoes, halved

2 medium cloves garlic or 1 teaspoon bottled minced garlic

2 tablespoons balsamic vinegar

1 teaspoon salt-free Italian seasoning

⅛ teaspoon pepper

1 tablespoon plus 1½ teaspoons shredded or grated Parmesan cheese

Preheat oven to 400° F.

Spray a large baking sheet with olive oil spray. Arrange zucchini, squash, carrot, onion, asparagus, tomatoes (cut side up), and garlic in a single layer. Lightly spray tops with olive oil spray.

Bake without stirring for 20 to 25 minutes, or until tender.

Put half the vegetables in a food processor or blender. Process for 1 to 1½ minutes, or until mixture is desired consistency (almost smooth but with some texture is recommended). Put mixture in a medium bowl. Repeat.

Stir in vinegar, Italian seasoning, and pepper. Sprinkle with Parmesan.

COOK'S TIP

You can serve leftovers chilled or reheated. To reheat, put leftovers in a microwave-safe dish and heat, uncovered, on 100 percent power (high) until warm.

(PER SERVING)

Calories 31

Protein 2 g

Carbohydrates 6 g

Cholesterol 1 mg

Total Fat 1 g

Saturated 0 g

Polyunsaturated 0 g

Monounsaturated 0 g

Fiber 2 g

Sodium 25 mg

Italian Quiche in Phyllo Shells

- Serves 20; 1 shell per serving
- Preparation time: 10 minutes
- Thawing time: 10 minutes
- Cooking time: 14 to 15 minutes

Delight your guests with these mini morsels, made with convenient frozen phyllo shells. If you have time, though, you might want to make your own shells. Then you'll have enough to make Cinnamon Sugar Phyllo Snacks (our Cook's Tips, below, will tell you how).

20 frozen phyllo shells

4 ounces low-fat Italian turkey sausage

Egg substitute equivalent to 2 eggs, or 2 large eggs

¼ cup fat-free milk

1 green onion, chopped

2 tablespoons chopped black olives

2 tablespoons shredded or grated Parmesan cheese

¼ teaspoon dried oregano, crumbled

Preheat oven to 375° F. Put phyllo shells on a non-stick baking sheet and let thaw at room temperature for 10 minutes.

Meanwhile, remove casing from sausage. In a small nonstick skillet over medium-high heat, cook sausage for 4 to 5 minutes, or until no longer pink, stirring occasionally to break up. Put in a colander and rinse with hot water to remove excess fat; drain well.

In a medium bowl, whisk together remaining ingredients. Stir in sausage, then pour mixture evenly into phyllo shells.

Bake for 10 minutes, or until centers are set.

COOK'S TIP ON MAKING PHYLLO SHELLS

Phyllo shells are simple to make. Preheat the oven to 375° F. Lightly spray 20 mini-muffin cups with olive oil spray. Put three 12 x 16-inch sheets of phyllo on a large cutting board. Lightly spray top sheet with olive oil spray. With kitchen scissors, cut phyllo into twenty 3-inch squares. You'll have strips of phyllo about 1 inch wide remaining. (See Cook's Tip on Cinnamon Sugar

Phyllo Snacks for how to use the extra pieces.) Put one square of phyllo in each muffin cup, pressing gently into the cups with your fingers. To use with fillings that must be cooked, bake shells for 5 minutes, or until lightly golden. To use with no-cook fillings, such as Mini Vegetable Cheese Balls on page 39, bake them for 10 to 13 minutes, or until golden brown. Remove from muffin tins and cool on a rack before filling.

For phyllo shells to use with sweet fillings, spray dough with butter-flavor vegetable oil spray. Combine 1 tablespoon sugar and ¼ teaspoon ground cinnamon; sprinkle on shells. Bake for 10 to 13 minutes, cool, and fill with fresh fruit, fat-free or low-fat yogurt, or pudding made with fat-free milk.

COOK'S TIP ON CINNAMON SUGAR PHYLLO SNACKS

Cut three 1-inch strips of phyllo crosswise into 4 pieces each and put the strips on a medium baking sheet. Lightly spray the tops with butter-flavor vegetable oil spray. Combine ½ teaspoon sugar and ⅛ teaspoon ground cinnamon; sprinkle over the phyllo. Bake at 375° F for 6 to 8 minutes, or until golden.

(PER SERVING)
Calories 77
Protein 5 g
Carbohydrates 5 g
Cholesterol 5 mg
Total Fat 4 g
  Saturated 1 g
  Polyunsaturated —
  Monounsaturated —
Fiber 0 g
Sodium 179 mg

Turkey Potstickers

- Serves 10; 3 dumplings per serving
- Preparation time: 20 minutes
- Cooking time: 13 to 17 minutes

Traditional Asian pan-fried dumplings are known as potstickers because they tend to stick to the bottom of the pot. This recipe calls for a nonstick skillet, so the potstickers will be brown on the bottom without sticking.

Filling

½ pound lean ground skinless turkey breast

2 tablespoons chopped pimiento, drained

2 tablespoons chopped water chestnuts, rinsed and drained

1 tablespoon reduced-sodium teriyaki sauce

1 teaspoon bottled minced garlic or 2 medium cloves garlic, minced

½ teaspoon grated gingerroot or ⅛ teaspoon ground ginger

■ ■ ■

30 wonton wrappers

1 tablespoon acceptable vegetable oil

1½ cups water

½ cup low-sodium chicken broth

⅓ cup plus 1 tablespoon sweet-and-sour sauce

In a medium bowl, combine all filling ingredients, using your hands or a spoon.

Put as many wonton wrappers as you can in one layer on wax paper. Spoon about 1½ teaspoons filling down center of each wrapper. With a pastry brush or your finger, lightly moisten two adjoining edges of each wrapper with water. Fold wrappers diagonally in half over filling (corner to corner, creating a triangle), pressing moistened edges of wrapper to dry edges to seal. Set dumplings aside. Repeat with remaining wrappers and filling.

Heat a 12-inch nonstick skillet over medium-high heat. Add oil and swirl to coat bottom of skillet. Place dumplings crowded together in a single layer with folded edge down and opposite end (point of triangle) pointing up slightly. Cook dumplings for 1 to 2 minutes, or until folded edges are golden brown. (Don't turn dumplings.)

Add water and broth. Reduce heat to medium-low and cook, covered, for 8 to 10 minutes, or until filling is cooked through (cut open a dumpling to check). Un-cover and cook over medium-high heat for 2 to 3 min-utes, or until dumplings are brown on bottom (don't stir, but check occasionally so they don't burn).

Serve dumplings with browned area showing. Serve with sweet-and-sour sauce on the side.

COOK'S TIP

If you don't have a 12-inch skillet, use two smaller skil-lets (two 10-inch skillets work fine). Cook dumplings in a single layer so they'll brown nicely.

COOK'S TIP ON GARLIC

If you have some sprouting garlic in your kitchen, you can still use it. If the sprouting garlic is in the supermar-ket, bypass it—its shelf life has reached an end.

(PER SERVING)

Calories 130
Protein 8 g
Carbohydrates 19 g
Cholesterol 13 mg
Total Fat 2 g
  Saturated 0 g
   Polyunsaturated 1 g
   Monounsaturated 0 g
Fiber 0 g
Sodium 349 mg

Stacked Mushroom Nachos

- Serves 8; 2 nachos per serving
- Preparation time: 15 minutes
- Cooking time: 10 minutes

These nachos use mushrooms instead of high-fat fried chips as their base. Plan on having plenty around—they disappear quickly!

16 large fresh mushrooms, stems removed

Olive oil spray

¼ teaspoon chili powder

⅓ cup fat-free refried beans

8 cherry tomatoes, quartered

⅓ cup fat-free or reduced-fat shredded Cheddar cheese

16 black olive slices

Preheat oven to 350° F.

Put mushrooms stem side down on a nonstick baking sheet. Lightly spray tops with olive oil spray. Sprinkle with chili powder. Turn mushrooms over.

Spread 1 teaspoon beans over cavity of each mushroom. Place a cherry tomato quarter cut side up on beans; slightly press tomato into beans to secure it. Sprinkle with cheese and top with olive slices.

Bake for 10 minutes, or until warmed through.

(PER SERVING)

Calories 31

Protein 3 g

Carbohydrates 4 g

Cholesterol 0 mg

Total Fat 0 g

  Saturated 0 g

  Polyunsaturated 0 g

  Monounsaturated 0 g

Fiber 1 g

Sodium 95 mg

Morning Energy Drink

Serves 4; 1 cup per serving ∎
Preparation time: 10 minutes ∎

Get up and go with this satisfying breakfast drink. For a frosty presentation, put empty glasses in the freezer just before you prepare the drink.

1½ cups fat-free nondairy soy beverage or fat-free milk

1 cup frozen peaches (keep frozen) (10 ounces)

1 cup strawberries, stems removed (about 7 ounces)

1 cup carrot juice

1 small banana (4 ounces)

2 tablespoons wheat germ or oat bran (optional)

2 tablespoons honey

Put all ingredients in a blender. Blend until smooth, about 1 minute.

MORNING ENERGY "SOUP"

For a change, serve this dish as a cold soup for breakfast. Pour 1 cup into a bowl and top with about ¼ cup of your favorite fat-free or low-fat cereal, such as wheat biscuits. (Calories 208; Protein 5 g; Carbohydrates 50 g; Cholesterol 0 mg; Total Fat 1 g; Saturated 0 g; Polyunsaturated 0 g; Monounsaturated 0 g; Fiber 4 g; Sodium 100 mg)

(PER SERVING)

Calories 182

Protein 4 g

Carbohydrates 44 g

Cholesterol 0 mg

Total Fat 0 g

  Saturated 0 g

  Polyunsaturated 0 g

  Monounsaturated 0 g

Fiber 3 g

Sodium 48 mg

Pineapple Shakes

- Serves 4; 1 cup per serving
- Preparation time: 5 minutes

Sample a taste of the tropics when you make this creamy shake. If you'd rather, you can freeze it for a semisoft treat.

6-ounce can pineapple juice

8-ounce container fat-free or low-fat vanilla yogurt (1 cup)

1-pound bag frozen mixed fruit or raspberries (partially thawed for shake)

¼ cup confectioners' sugar

Put all ingredients in a blender in order listed. Blend until smooth (if using raspberries, pour blended mixture into a strainer and press through, using back of a spoon). Pour into four glasses.

ORANGE SHAKES

Replace pineapple juice with orange juice, mixed fruit with strawberries, and sugar with a medium banana (5 to 6 ounces). (Calories 138; Protein 4 g; Carbohydrates 32 g; Cholesterol 1 mg; Total Fat 0 g; Saturated 0 g; Polyunsaturated 0 g; Monounsaturated 0 g; Fiber 3 g; Sodium 34 mg)

VARIATION

(PER SERVING)

Calories 147

Protein 3 g

Carbohydrates 34 g

Cholesterol 1 mg

Total Fat 0 g

Saturated 0 g

Polyunsaturated 0 g

Monounsaturated 0 g

Fiber 2 g

Sodium 32 mg

To change this recipe from shakes to dessert, seal the mixture in an airtight freezer bag and freeze for about 1 hour. Let it stand for a few minutes to soften slightly before serving. Serves 8; ½ cup per serving.

Strawberry Mint Spritzer

Serves 6; 1 cup per serving ■
Preparation time: 5 minutes ■

Ideal as a refreshing spritzer for brunch or on a hot summer day, this sparkling drink will be like a smoothie if you vary the proportion of strawberry mixture and sparkling water.

6 fresh mint leaves

1 pound strawberries (about 2 cups)

½ cup sugar

Grated zest of 1 medium lime (about 1 teaspoon)

2 tablespoons lime juice (1 to 2 medium limes)

4 cups club soda, sparkling water, or seltzer

6 lime wedges (optional)

6 mint sprigs (optional)

Chop mint leaves into very small pieces.

Stem and halve strawberries. Put in a food processor or blender and process until smooth.

Add sugar, lime zest, lime juice, and chopped mint leaves; process until blended.

To serve, pour ⅓ cup strawberry mixture and ⅔ cup club soda into each glass; add ice and stir. Garnish with a lime wedge and mint sprig.

STRAWBERRY MINT SMOOTHIE

For a smoothie-like drink, use equal amounts of strawberry mixture and club soda. Serves 4; 1 cup per serving. (Calories 132; Protein 1 g; Carbohydrates 34 g; Cholesterol 0 mg; Total Fat 0 g; Saturated 0 g; Polyunsaturated 0 g; Monounsaturated 0 g; Fiber 3 g; Sodium 34 mg)

(PER SERVING)

Calories 88

Protein 1 g

Carbohydrates 22 g

Cholesterol 0 mg

Total Fat 0 g

　Saturated 0 g

　Polyunsaturated 0 g

　Monounsaturated 0 g

Fiber 2 g

Sodium 36 mg

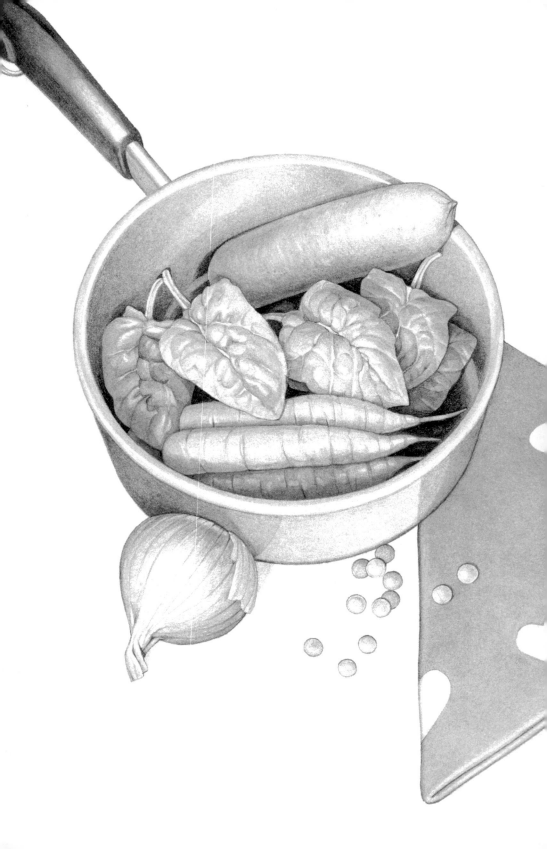

SOUPS

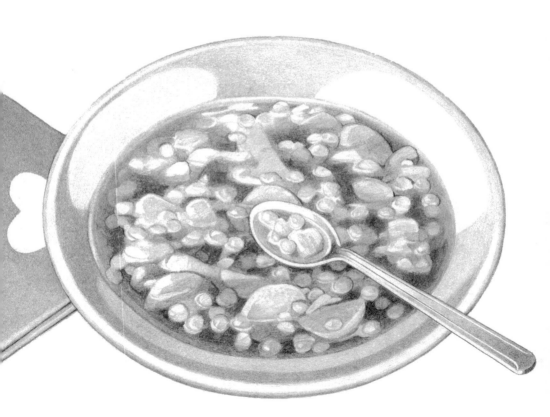

■ ■ ■

Butternut Squash Soup

Tomato Basil Soup

Corn and Chicken Chowder

   Corn and Cheddar Chowder

Turkey Tortilla Soup

Spinach Lentil Soup

Meatball Soup with Sun-Dried
Tomatoes and Swiss Chard

Pizza Soup

   Spaghetti Soup

White Bean and Pasta Soup

   Mixed Bean and Pasta Soup

Creamy Mushroom Barley Soup

Chilled Strawberry Orange Soup

■ ■ ■

Butternut Squash Soup

Serves 6; ¼ cup per serving ■
Preparation time: 10 minutes ■
Cooking time: 10 to 12 minutes ■

Butternut squash gives a velvety texture to this soup. Every spoonful contains colorful bits of vegetables and fresh dill.

1 teaspoon light margarine

2 medium carrots, diced (about 1½ cups)

¼ cup frozen chopped onion or ½ medium onion, diced

1 teaspoon bottled minced garlic or 2 medium cloves garlic, minced

4 cups low-sodium chicken broth

½ cup frozen no-salt-added whole-kernel corn

½ cup frozen butternut squash, thawed

½ cup water

⅓ cup all-purpose flour

1 tablespoon snipped fresh dillweed or 1 teaspoon dried, crumbled

Heat a large saucepan over medium-high heat. Cook margarine, carrots, onion, and garlic for 2 to 3 minutes, or until vegetables are tender, stirring occasionally.

Add broth, corn, and squash. Increase heat to high and bring to a boil, 4 to 5 minutes, stirring occasionally.

In a small bowl, stir together water and flour. Add to soup and cook over high heat for 3 to 4 minutes, or until mixture is thickened and bubbly.

Add dillweed and cook for 30 to 60 seconds, stirring occasionally.

COOK'S TIP ON FROZEN BUTTERNUT SQUASH

To avoid wasting half a package of frozen butternut squash, cut the package in half with a sturdy serrated knife. Freeze one half in an airtight plastic bag for later use—perhaps to thaw and swirl together with mashed potatoes for a fun and different side dish.

(PER SERVING)

Calories 88

Protein 4 g

Carbohydrates 16 g

Cholesterol 1 mg

Total Fat 1 g

  Saturated 0 g

  Polyunsaturated 0 g

  Monounsaturated 0 g

Fiber 2 g

Sodium 87 mg

Tomato Basil Soup

- Serves 4; ¾ cup per serving
- Preparation time: 5 minutes
- Cooking time: 18 minutes

Enjoy this refreshing, light soup year-round. The cilantro or parsley gives the soup a fresh taste even when basil is out of season.

14.5-ounce can no-salt-added diced tomatoes, undrained

14.5-ounce can low-sodium chicken broth

2 tablespoons fresh basil or 2 teaspoons dried, crumbled

1 teaspoon sugar

¾ teaspoon very low sodium or low-sodium Worcestershire sauce

⅛ teaspoon crushed red pepper flakes (optional)

¼ to ½ cup snipped fresh cilantro or parsley

2 teaspoons extra-virgin olive oil

¼ teaspoon salt

In a medium saucepan, combine undrained tomatoes, broth, basil, sugar, Worcestershire sauce, and red pepper; bring to a boil, covered, over high heat. Reduce heat and simmer, uncovered, for 15 minutes. Remove from heat.

Stir in remaining ingredients.

COOK'S TIP

If you prepare this dish in advance, add the cilantro, oil, and salt after reheating.

(PER SERVING)

Calories 61

Protein 2 g

Carbohydrates 7 g

Cholesterol 0 mg

Total Fat 3 g

　Saturated 0 g

　Polyunsaturated 0 g

　Monounsaturated 2 g

Fiber 2 g

Sodium 188 mg

Corn and Chicken Chowder

Serves 3; 1¼ cups per serving ■
Preparation time: 10 minutes ■
Cooking time: 11 to 12 minutes ■

Simple to prepare, this chowder has a rich flavor and an interesting texture that make it enormously satisfying. Serve it with a crisp salad plus fruit for dessert, and you have a delectable light dinner.

14-ounce can cream-style corn

1 cup frozen ~~no-salt-added whole-kernel corn~~ *mixed vegetables*

1 cup fat-free milk

5-ounce can all-white chicken packed in water, drained

2 tablespoons minced red or green bell pepper or 2 tablespoons bottled roasted red bell pepper or bottled cherry peppers, rinsed and drained

¼ teaspoon dried thyme, crumbled

⅛ teaspoon pepper (white preferred) (omit if using cherry peppers)

In a medium saucepan, combine both corns, milk, and chicken. Heat over low heat for 5 minutes, stirring occasionally.

Stir in remaining ingredients. Increase heat to medium-low and cook for 3 to 4 minutes, or until soup just begins to simmer. Simmer for 3 minutes, or until hot.

Corn and Cheddar Chowder

Reduce cream-style corn to ½ can, and increase whole-kernel corn to 1½ cups. Substitute ½ to ¾ cup grated reduced-fat Cheddar cheese for the chicken. (Calories 219; Protein 14 g; Carbohydrates 34 g; Cholesterol 17 mg; Total Fat 5 g; Saturated 3 g; Polyunsaturated 1 g; Monounsaturated 2 g; Fiber 3 g; Sodium 383 mg)

Cook's Tip

For additional richness without added fat, add ¾ cup frozen mashed potatoes to the soup along with the corns, milk, and chicken.

(PER SERVING)

Calories 250

Protein 21 g

Carbohydrates 40 g

Cholesterol 41 mg

Total Fat 3 g

   Saturated 1 g

    Polyunsaturated 1 g

     Monounsaturated 1 g

Fiber 3 g

Sodium 455 mg

Turkey Tortilla Soup

- Serves 4; 1½ cups per serving
- Preparation time: 10 minutes
- Cooking time: 17 minutes

For a unique presentation, place a shaped baked tortilla half in each bowl of this zippy soup. Use leftover turkey from the holidays, or for a grilled turkey tortilla soup, use leftover grilled turkey from the Grilled Turkey Cutlets with Pineapple—without the pineapple, of course (page 181).

2 6-inch corn tortillas

Vegetable oil spray

¼ teaspoon chili powder

1 tablespoon light margarine

½ cup frozen chopped onion or 1 medium onion, chopped

½ cup chopped carrot

1 Anaheim pepper, seeded and chopped

14.5-ounce can no-salt-added stewed tomatoes

2 cups low-sodium chicken broth

2 cups water

8-ounce can no-salt-added tomato sauce (1 cup)

1 cup diced skinless cooked turkey (6 ounces)

1 tablespoon ground cumin

1 teaspoon chili powder

¼ cup shredded nonfat or low-fat Cheddar cheese (about 1 ounce)

(PER SERVING)

Calories 188

Protein 17 g

Carbohydrates 17 g

Cholesterol 28 mg

Total Fat 6 g

  Saturated 1 g

  Polyunsaturated 2 g

  Monounsaturated 2 g

Fiber 4 g

Sodium 214 mg

Preheat oven to 350° F.

Cut tortillas in half. Lightly spray tops with vegetable oil spray. Sprinkle with ¼ teaspoon chili powder. Place each tortilla half cut side down (cut side touching bottom of tin, framing a "bottomless" cup) in a muffin cup, bending tortillas slightly to fit.

Bake for 5 minutes, or until crisp. Remove muffin pan from oven, leaving tortillas in muffin cups; set aside.

Meanwhile, in a large stockpot, melt margarine over medium-high heat. Stir in onions, carrots, and pepper. Cook for 2 to 3 minutes, or until vegetables are tender, stirring occasionally.

Stir in remaining ingredients except cheese; bring to a boil over high heat. Reduce heat and simmer, uncovered, for 10 minutes, or until flavors are blended, stirring occasionally.

To serve, place a tortilla piece cut side down in each bowl. Ladle soup into bowls and sprinkle with cheese.

Spinach Lentil Soup

Serves 8; 1½ cups per serving ■
Preparation time: 10 minutes ■
Cooking time: 40 to 45 minutes ■

Soups with vegetables and lentils or other legumes are satisfying and nutritious—wonderful when you want to eat well but not overindulge.

4 ounces low-fat turkey kielbasa, cut in bite-size pieces, or low-fat ground sausage

½ cup frozen chopped onion or 1 medium onion, minced

1 medium carrot, finely chopped

¼ teaspoon crushed red pepper flakes

6 cups water

2 cups low-sodium chicken broth

1 cup red lentils, sorted for stones and shriveled lentils and rinsed

10 ounces fresh spinach

1 cup cooked rice (optional)

Put sausage in a 4-quart stockpot or Dutch oven over high heat (if using ground sausage, break it up with a wooden spoon or fork as it cooks).

Add onion, carrot, and red pepper flakes. Cook until onion is translucent, about 3 minutes.

Add water, broth, and lentils; bring to a boil over high heat. Reduce heat and simmer for 25 to 30 minutes, or until lentils are tender, stirring occasionally.

Meanwhile, cut spinach into strips about ½ inch wide. Add spinach and rice to soup and cook for 5 minutes.

COOK'S TIP

If you heat leftover soup, expect the spinach to turn light green.

(PER SERVING)

Calories 124

Protein 11 g

Carbohydrates 18 g

Cholesterol 9 mg

Total Fat 2 g

   Saturated 0 g

    Polyunsaturated 0 g

    Monounsaturated 0 g

Fiber 9 g

Sodium 197 mg

Meatball Soup with Sun-Dried Tomatoes and Swiss Chard

- Serves 4; 1½ cups per serving
- Preparation time: 20 minutes
- Cooking time: 12 to 15 minutes

If you've never cooked Swiss chard before, here's your chance. It adds lots of both flavor and nutrients to this filling soup. With a little practice, you can roll the meatballs in only about five minutes.

Vegetable oil spray

Meatballs

½ pound lean ground beef

¼ cup plain dry bread crumbs

Egg substitute equivalent to 1 egg, or 1 large egg

2 teaspoons chopped fresh savory or ½ teaspoon dried, crumbled, or 2 teaspoons chopped fresh oregano or ½ teaspoon dried, crumbled

½ teaspoon salt-free Italian seasoning, crumbled

■ ■ ■

6 cups low-sodium chicken broth

½ cup frozen chopped onion or 1 medium onion, chopped

2 tablespoons dry-packed sun-dried tomatoes, cut into thin strips, or 1 tablespoon no-salt-added tomato paste

2 tablespoons salt-free Italian seasoning, crumbled

1 teaspoon bottled minced garlic or 2 medium cloves garlic, minced

⅛ teaspoon pepper

¼ cup dried small pasta, such as ditalini

4 cups Swiss chard leaves, cut into ½-inch strips (about 8 ounces or 1 bunch), or 10-ounce package frozen chopped spinach, thawed

1 tablespoon plus 1 teaspoon shredded or grated Parmesan cheese

Spray a broiler pan with vegetable oil spray; set aside. Preheat broiler.

For meatballs, combine ingredients in a medium bowl, using your hands to mix together lightly. With your hands, roll mixture into about 45 tiny meatballs, about 1 teaspoon each. Put meatballs on broiler pan.

Broil meatballs about 6 inches from heat for 3 to 4 minutes, or until brown on top. Turn meatballs over and broil for 3 to 4 minutes, or until brown.

While meatballs are broiling, put broth, onions, tomatoes, 2 tablespoons Italian seasoning, garlic, and pepper in a large stockpot; bring to a boil over high heat.

Add pasta and reduce heat to medium-high. Cook for 4 to 5 minutes, or until pasta is tender, stirring occasionally.

Meanwhile, if using spinach, drain and squeeze out all liquid.

Add meatballs and chard to broth mixture; reduce heat and simmer for 2 minutes, stirring occasionally.

To serve, ladle soup into bowls and sprinkle with Parmesan.

TIME-SAVER

To make this soup even more quickly, add 6 ounces of cooked lean ground beef or turkey (rinsed in hot water after cooking) instead of making meatballs. (Start with 8 ounces raw beef or turkey.) If you are grilling hamburgers up to five days before making the soup, grill two extra burgers (each 4 ounces before cooking), cut them into ½-inch cubes, and refrigerate in an airtight plastic bag. When you make the soup, add the leftover hamburger cubes after the pasta is tender.

COOK'S TIP ON SMALL PASTA

You will love how quickly tiny pastas cook. Also known as pastinas, these include acini di pepe, which are small nuggets, and ditalini, which are slightly larger and resemble short tubes. The next time you are at the grocery store, look for different shapes to keep on hand for soup or a quick side dish.

(PER SERVING)

Calories 225

Protein 24 g

Carbohydrates 19 g

Cholesterol 38 mg

Total Fat 7 g

  Saturated 2 g

  Polyunsaturated 0 g

  Monounsaturated 2 g

Fiber 2 g

Sodium 473 mg

Pizza Soup

- Serves 4; 1½ cups per serving
- Preparation time: 5 minutes
- Cooking time: 5 minutes

You can make this robust soup in less time than it takes to have a pizza delivered. The soup is a lot more nutritious—and costs less too.

3 ounces Italian sausage (casing removed)

¾ cup frozen chopped green bell pepper or 1 medium green bell pepper, chopped

½ cup frozen chopped onion or 1 medium onion, chopped

8 ounces presliced fresh mushrooms

4 cups water

16-ounce can no-salt-added chick-peas

14.5-ounce can no-salt-added crushed tomatoes

1 teaspoon dried basil, crumbled

½ teaspoon dried oregano, crumbled

½ teaspoon crushed red pepper flakes

In a 4-quart stockpot, heat sausage over medium heat, breaking it into small pieces with a spoon as it cooks. Cook for 5 minutes.

Add bell pepper, onion, and mushrooms. Increase heat to high. Cook until vegetables have softened, about 5 minutes, stirring occasionally.

Add remaining ingredients. Bring to a boil and serve.

(PER SERVING)

Calories 231

Protein 12 g

Carbohydrates 27 g

Cholesterol 16 mg

Total Fat 9 g

Saturated 2 g

Polyunsaturated —

Monounsaturated —

Fiber 7 g

Sodium 188 mg

SPAGHETTI SOUP

Break 2 to 3 ounces dried vermicelli into small pieces. Prepare using package directions, omitting salt and oil. Drain and add to soup. Lots of pasta makes a very thick, stewy soup; less just adds a nice "chew." Serves 5; 1⅓ cups per serving. (Calories 235; Protein 11 g; Carbohydrates 32 g; Cholesterol 13 mg; Total Fat 7 g; Saturated 2 g; Polyunsaturated 1 g; Monounsaturated 2 g; Fiber 6 g; Sodium 151 mg)

White Bean and Pasta Soup

Serves 4; 1 cup per serving ■
Preparation time: 5 minutes ■
Cooking time: 10 minutes ■

For a taste of Italy in minutes, prepare this simple soup. Serve with a hearty peasant bread.

15-ounce can no-salt-added Great Northern beans, rinsed and drained

3 cups low-sodium chicken broth

1 cup no-salt-added canned diced tomatoes, drained

½ teaspoon dried oregano, crumbled

½ cup miniature pasta shells

1 tablespoon plus 1 teaspoon shredded or grated Parmesan cheese

In a large saucepan, combine beans, broth, tomatoes, and oregano. Bring to a boil over medium heat.

Stir in pasta. Cook, partially covered, for 7 minutes, or until pasta is just cooked through.

To serve, ladle into soup bowls and sprinkle with cheese.

MIXED BEAN AND PASTA SOUP

Substitute a can of rinsed and drained mixed beans (no salt added preferred) for the Great Northern beans and add 1 cup no-salt-added frozen green beans to the mix. Serves 5; 1 cup per serving. (Calories 155; Protein 9 g; Carbohydrates 26 g; Cholesterol 2 mg; Total Fat 2 g; Saturated 0 g; Polyunsaturated 0 g; Monounsaturated 0 g; Fiber 6 g; Sodium 100 mg)

COOK'S TIP

If you have soup left over, the pasta will tend to absorb the liquid. When reheating the soup, add enough water, tomato liquid from draining the tomatoes, or chicken broth to make a soupy consistency.

(PER SERVING)

Calories 177

Protein 11 g

Carbohydrates 29 g

Cholesterol 2 mg

Total Fat 2 g

  Saturated 0 g

  Polyunsaturated 0 g

  Monounsaturated 0 g

Fiber 6 g

Sodium 124 mg

Creamy Mushroom Barley Soup

- Serves 9; 1½ cups per serving
- Preparation time: 10 minutes
- Cooking time: 30 minutes

Buying the mushrooms presliced will hurry things along in this recipe. Another handy convenience food: frozen chopped onions.

¾ cup very hot tap water

½ to 1 ounce dried porcini mushrooms

1 tablespoon acceptable vegetable oil

½ cup frozen chopped onion or 1 medium onion, minced

1 or 2 medium carrots, diced

16 to 20 ounces presliced fresh mushrooms

1¼ teaspoons dried thyme, crumbled

5 cups water

2 cups low-sodium chicken broth

⅓ cup uncooked quick-cooking barley

Pepper to taste

½ teaspoon salt

¾ cup fat-free milk

3 tablespoons all-purpose flour

1 to 2 tablespoons dry sherry (optional)

In a small bowl, combine ¾ cup hot water and dried mushrooms; set aside.

Heat a 4-quart stockpot over high heat. Add oil and swirl to coat bottom of pot. Cook onion and carrot for about 5 minutes, or until vegetables start to soften, stirring occasionally.

Stir in fresh mushrooms and thyme; cook for 5 minutes.

Stir in 5 cups water, broth, barley, and pepper; bring to a boil. Reduce heat and simmer, uncovered, for 10 minutes.

Meanwhile, drain dried mushrooms, adding soaking liquid to pot. Chop mushrooms; stir mushrooms and salt into pot.

In a jar with a tight-fitting lid, combine milk and flour. Cover and shake until completely blended. Add to soup; bring to a boil. Reduce heat and simmer for at least 2 minutes.

Stir in sherry.

(PER SERVING)

Calories 83

Protein 4 g

Carbohydrates 14 g

Cholesterol 1 mg

Total Fat 2 g

Saturated 0 g

Polyunsaturated 1 g

Monounsaturated 0 g

Fiber 2 g

Sodium 167 mg

Chilled Strawberry Orange Soup

Serves 6; ⅔ cup per serving ■

Preparation time: 5 minutes ■

Chilling time: 1 hour, if using fresh strawberries ■

Serve this chilled fruit soup as a light summer appetizer or with your favorite sandwich or salad.

1 pound fresh or frozen unsweetened
   strawberries, slightly thawed
   (about 1 pint)

1½ cups orange juice (4 to 5 medium
   oranges)

¼ cup sugar

2 tablespoons lime juice (optional)
   (1 to 2 medium limes)

1 teaspoon grated gingerroot

In a food processor or blender, process all ingredients until smooth.

If using fresh strawberries, cover and refrigerate for 1 hour to chill thoroughly. If using frozen strawberries, serve immediately or cover and refrigerate until needed.

COOK'S TIP

Serve this soup within 24 hours for peak flavor.

(PER SERVING)

Calories 83

Protein 1 g

Carbohydrates 20 g

Cholesterol 0 mg

Total Fat 0 g

  Saturated 0 g

  Polyunsaturated 0 g

  Monounsaturated 0 g

Fiber 2 g

Sodium 2 mg

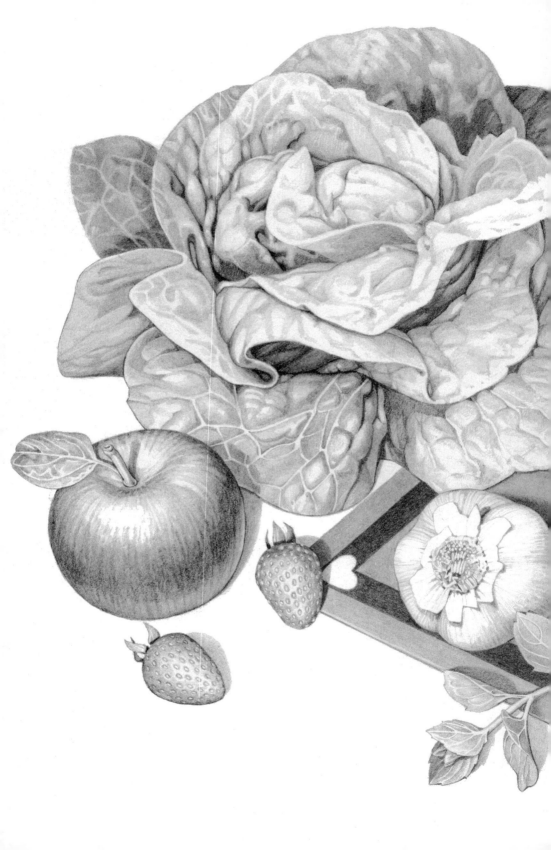

SALADS AND SALAD DRESSINGS

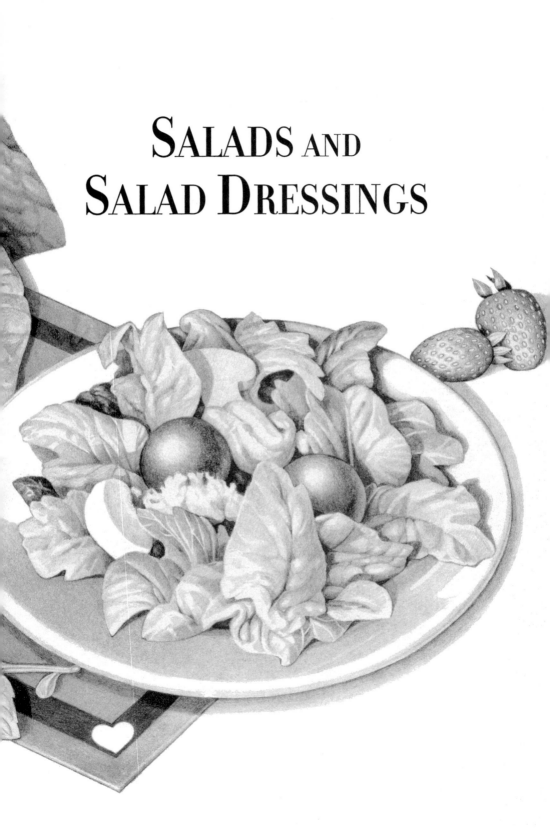

■ ■ ■

Mixed Salad Greens and Fruit with Fresh Strawberry Vinaigrette

Green and Petite Pea Salad with Feta

Mimosa Salad

Warm Napa Slaw

   Warm Napa Slaw with Chicken

Cabbage Slaw with Roasted Peanut Oil Dressing

Greek Cucumber Salad

Peach Fans on Blackberry-Lime Sauce

   Pear Fans on Raspberry Sauce

Pear and Goat Cheese Salad

Mixed Fruit Salad with Mango Dressing

Strawberry-Mango Salsa

   Peach Salsa

Orange-Pineapple Gelatin Salad

   Lime-Pineapple Gelatin Salad

German Potato Salad

   Mexican Potato Salad

Barley and Vegetable Salad

Italian Bean and Tuna Salad

Southwestern Chicken Salad

Asian Chicken and Wild Rice Salad

Chicken and Grapefruit Salad

Beef Salad with Vinaigrette Dressing

   Beef Salad with Horseradish Dressing

Thai Beef Salad

Vegetarian Taco Salad

Fresh Herb Couscous Salad

Orzo Salad with Green Peas and Artichokes

Wheat Berry Salad

Far East Dressing

   Far East Chicken Salad

Pepper Dijon Dressing

   Tarragon Dijon Dressing

Roasted Red Bell Pepper Dressing

■ ■ ■

Mixed Salad Greens and Fruit with Fresh Strawberry Vinaigrette

Serves 4; 2¼ cups per serving ■
Preparation time: 10 minutes ■

Serve this brilliantly colored salad of mixed salad greens, blueberries, mandarin oranges, and pears with Farmers' Market Stovetop Casserole (page 255).

Strawberry Vinaigrette

2 cups whole strawberries, stemmed

¼ cup sugar

¼ cup raspberry vinegar

■ ■ ■

8 ounces mixed salad greens (about 8 cups)

½ cup red onion, thinly sliced (about 2 ounces)

11-ounce can mandarin oranges in water or light syrup, well drained

1 large pear, thinly sliced (about 8 ounces)

1 cup blueberries or quartered strawberries

3 tablespoons sliced almonds, dry-roasted (¾ ounce)

In a food processor or blender, process vinaigrette ingredients until smooth.

Arrange salad greens on a serving platter; drizzle with dressing. Top with remaining ingredients.

Serve immediately.

Cook's Tip on Dry-Roasting Nuts

To bring out the flavor, roast nuts in an ungreased skillet over medium heat for 1 to 5 minutes, stirring frequently, or in a shallow baking pan at 350° F for 10 to 15 minutes, stirring occasionally. Watch carefully; the nuts can burn easily.

(PER SERVING)

Calories 187

Protein 3 g

Carbohydrates 40 g

Cholesterol 0 mg

Total Fat 3 g

  Saturated 0 g

    Polyunsaturated 1 g

    Monounsaturated 2 g

Fiber 7 g

Sodium 10 mg

Green and Petite Pea Salad with Feta

- Serves 4; 1¼ cups per serving
- Preparation time: 10 minutes

Remember those 24-hour layered salads? This speedier dish is more sophisticated and healthful.

4 cups torn mixed salad greens
(about 6 ounces)

1 cup frozen petite green peas,
thawed (about 4 ounces)

1 ounce red onion, thinly sliced

¼ cup fat-free or light ranch-style
salad dressing

1 tablespoon fat-free milk

2 ounces tomato-basil or plain feta
cheese, rinsed and crumbled, or
shredded fat-free or reduced-fat
Cheddar cheese

Freshly ground pepper to taste

In a medium bowl, combine salad greens, peas, and onion.

In a small bowl, whisk together salad dressing and milk until smooth.

To serve, spoon dressing mixture over salad, then sprinkle with feta and pepper. Toss gently. Sprinkle with additional pepper.

COOK'S TIP ON THAWING VEGETABLES

To thaw frozen vegetables quickly, put them in a colander and run them under cold water for 15 to 20 seconds; drain well.

(PER SERVING)

Calories 100

Protein 5 g

Carbohydrates 13 g

Cholesterol 13 mg

Total Fat 3 g

  Saturated 2 g

  Polyunsaturated 0 g

  Monounsaturated 1 g

Fiber 3 g

Sodium 341 mg

Mimosa Salad

Serves 4; 1¼ cups per serving ■
Preparation time: 10 minutes ■
Cooking time: 20 to 25 minutes ■

The different colors, shapes, and textures of just a few ingredients combine here for a simple, unusual salad.

4 large eggs

4 cups torn red-leaf lettuce

½ cup fat-free or light Thousand Island salad dressing

Paprika

Hard boil eggs.

Meanwhile, arrange 1 cup lettuce on each of four salad plates.

Drizzle each serving with 2 tablespoons dressing. Refrigerate.

When eggs are cooked, peel and cut each in half lengthwise. Remove yolks; discard all but 2 yolk halves.

To assemble, grate white of 1 egg and half of ½ yolk over each salad. Sprinkle with paprika.

(PER SERVING)

Calories 76

Protein 5 g

Carbohydrates 11 g

Cholesterol 53 mg

Total Fat 1 g

   Saturated 0 g

   Polyunsaturated 0 g

   Monounsaturated 0 g

Fiber 1 g

Sodium 375 mg

Warm Napa Slaw

- Serves 6; 1 cup per serving
- Preparation time: 15 minutes
- Cooking time: 7 minutes

This versatile Asian-flavored slaw can be as mild or as spicy as you like. Use it as a vegetable or a salad, or add chicken for a main dish.

6 cups slivered cabbage (napa preferred)

Dressing

1 tablespoon acceptable vegetable oil

2 tablespoons sesame seeds

1 bunch green onions, sliced (about 6)

1 teaspoon bottled minced garlic or 2 medium cloves garlic, minced

¼ cup low-sodium chicken broth or water

2 tablespoons vinegar (rice vinegar preferred)

1 to 1½ teaspoons light soy sauce

⅛ teaspoon crushed red pepper flakes, or to taste (optional)

1 teaspoon red hot sauce, or to taste (optional)

Put cabbage in a large serving bowl; set aside.

In a medium skillet, heat oil over high heat. Cook sesame seeds until they begin to brown, 1 minute, stirring constantly with a long-handled spoon (be careful—sesame seeds will "spit").

Add onions and garlic; cook for 1 minute, or until aromatic, stirring frequently.

Add remaining dressing ingredients except hot sauce; boil, uncovered, until liquid is reduced to about 3 tablespoons, 1 to 2 minutes. Pour over cabbage and drizzle with hot sauce.

WARM NAPA SLAW WITH CHICKEN

Prepare ⅔ cup uncooked rice using package directions, omitting salt and margarine. Meanwhile, cut 2 boneless, skinless chicken breast halves (about 4 ounces each) into slivers. Add them to the skillet after browning the sesame seeds and cooking the garlic and onions as directed above. Cook for 2 minutes, stirring constantly. Add the liquids and simmer until the chicken is cooked through, 2 to 3 minutes, stirring occasionally. Pour over cabbage and toss. Serve over rice. Serves 5 as a main dish, 1½ cups per serving. (Calories 259; Protein 18 g; Carbohydrates 30 g; Cholesterol 33 mg; Total Fat 8 g; Saturated 1 g; Polyunsaturated 3 g; Monounsaturated 1 g; Fiber 2 g; Sodium 233 mg)

COOK'S TIP ON CHINESE CABBAGE

There are many kinds of Chinese cabbage, and they seem to have multiple names. Don't worry. You can use Chinese cabbages interchangeably. They are generally milder than the hard-headed green cabbage, but even that, and savoy, can be used in this recipe.

Napa cabbage has pale, crinkly green leaves. It's easy to use: Just stack a bunch of the leaves and sliver by drawing your knife across the tip end and working back toward the root end. The closer you get to that end, the narrower you should cut the cabbage. Then you won't have large bites of tough stem.

(PER SERVING)

Calories 55
Protein 2 g
Carbohydrates 3 g
Cholesterol 0 mg
Total Fat 4 g
  Saturated 0 g
  Polyunsaturated 1 g
  Monounsaturated 1 g
Fiber 1 g
Sodium 135 mg

Cabbage Slaw with Roasted Peanut Oil Dressing

- Serves 8; ½ cup per serving
- Preparation time: 10 minutes

Just a small amount of roasted peanut oil gives a great amount of fragrance and flavor to the dressing for this crunchy salad. Serve with Tex-Mex or Asian food.

Slaw

5 cups shredded cabbage (about 10 ounces)

½ medium red bell pepper, thinly sliced

½ medium bell pepper, any color, thinly sliced

2 green onions, thinly sliced (about ¼ cup)

Roasted Peanut Oil Dressing

2 tablespoons lime juice (1 to 2 medium limes)

1 to 2 tablespoons snipped fresh cilantro

1 tablespoon honey

1 tablespoon roasted peanut oil

⅛ teaspoon salt

■ ■ ■

½ cup thinly sliced English cucumber (2 to 3 ounces) (optional)

In a medium bowl, stir together slaw ingredients.

In a small bowl, whisk together dressing ingredients. Stir into slaw mixture.

To serve, top with cucumber. Serve immediately or cover and refrigerate for up to four days.

COOK'S TIP ON ENGLISH CUCUMBERS

For longer storage life, remove the plastic wrapping before refrigerating the cucumbers.

(PER SERVING)

Calories 39

Protein 1 g

Carbohydrates 6 g

Cholesterol 0 mg

Total Fat 2 g

  Saturated 0 g

  Polyunsaturated 1 g

  Monounsaturated 1 g

Fiber 1 g

Sodium 47 mg

Greek Cucumber Salad

Serves 4; ½ cup per serving ■
Preparation time: 10 minutes ■

Cucumber salads are refreshing and easy. Maybe that's why they're found in so many cuisines. This one, with Greek overtones, uses fresh mint, but you can substitute fresh dillweed for a northern European flavor.

1 medium to large cucumber (8 to 10 ounces)

8-ounce container fat-free or low-fat plain yogurt or nonfat or light sour cream (1 cup)

¼ cup loosely packed chopped fresh mint or 1 tablespoon dried, crumbled

½ to 1 teaspoon bottled minced garlic or 1 or 2 medium cloves, chopped

⅛ to ¼ teaspoon salt

Peel cucumber if desired (if the skin seems waxy, you might want to peel it). Cut in half lengthwise. Scoop out seeds with a spoon; discard seeds. Slice cucumber into thin crescents.

In a medium bowl, stir together all ingredients.

Serve immediately or cover and refrigerate until needed.

TIME-SAVER

Removing the seeds from the cucumber makes the salad less watery. If you're in a hurry, you can omit this step.

(PER SERVING)

Calories 39

Protein 3 g

Carbohydrates 6 g

Cholesterol 1 mg

Total Fat 0 g

   Saturated 0 g

   Polyunsaturated 0 g

   Monounsaturated 0 g

Fiber 1 g

Sodium 180 mg

Peach Fans on Blackberry-Lime Sauce

- Serves 6; ¼ cup per serving
- Preparation time: 15 minutes
- Cooking time: 1 to 2 minutes
- Chilling time: 30 minutes to 24 hours

As a first course or light dessert, this dish is a showpiece!

¾ cup all-fruit seedless blackberry spread (about 8 ounces)

2 tablespoons lime juice (1 to 2 medium limes)

¼ teaspoon grated gingerroot (optional)

1¼ to 1½ pounds peaches (about 3½ cups)

18 whole medium strawberries with stems (about 1 pint)

In a small saucepan over medium-high heat, heat blackberry spread for 1 to 2 minutes, or until just melted, whisking constantly. Remove from heat.

Whisk in lime juice and gingerroot. Transfer to a medium bowl, cover, and refrigerate for 30 minutes to 24 hours.

Peel and slice peaches. Cut strawberries in half; if you cut the stem in half too, leaving half a stem on each piece, you'll have a prettier presentation.

To serve, spoon 2 tablespoons blackberry mixture onto center of a salad or dessert plate. Rotate plate to spread sauce to about a 6-inch circle. Alternating peaches and strawberries, arrange fruit accordion style. Repeat for each serving.

(PER SERVING)

Calories 138

Protein 1 g

Carbohydrates 35 g

Cholesterol 0 mg

Total Fat 0 g

  Saturated 0 g

  Polyunsaturated 0 g

  Monounsaturated 0 g

Fiber 3 g

Sodium 1 mg

PEAR FANS ON RASPBERRY SAUCE

Replace blackberry spread with seedless raspberry spread and omit lime juice. Replace peaches with two 8-ounce pears, and replace strawberries with 3 peeled kiwifruit, each cut lengthwise into sixths. (Calories 144; Protein 1 g; Carbohydrates 36 g; Cholesterol 0 mg; Total Fat 0 g; Saturated 0 g; Polyunsaturated 0 g; Monounsaturated 0 g; Fiber 3 g; Sodium 2 mg)

Pear and Goat Cheese Salad

Serves 8; 1 pear half per serving ■
Preparation time: 15 minutes ■
Cooking time: 5 minutes ■

Crunchy pecans and a mildly tart dressing enhance juicy, sweet pears topped with tangy goat cheese. For an out-of-the-ordinary light lunch, serve each person a double portion, along with a cup of soup.

¼ cup pecans (about 1 ounce)

3 to 4 cups chopped or torn salad greens

4 Bartlett or Anjou pears

2 ounces goat cheese or chèvre

2 tablespoons balsamic vinegar

1 teaspoon sugar (optional)

1 tablespoon olive oil

In a small skillet, dry-roast pecans over medium heat for 1 to 5 minutes, stirring frequently. Finely chop.

Meanwhile, arrange ½ cup salad greens on each of eight plates; set aside.

Cut pears in half lengthwise. With a melon baller, remove seeds and make a small, round cavity in each pear half.

Cut cheese into eight pieces; shape each into a ball. Roll in pecans and place one in each pear cavity. Arrange pears on lettuce.

Pour vinegar into a small bowl; add sugar, whisking until dissolved.

Add oil in a fine stream, whisking constantly until smooth. Drizzle evenly over pears; sprinkle with any remaining pecans.

(PER SERVING)

Calories 111

Protein 2 g

Carbohydrates 14 g

Cholesterol 3 mg

Total Fat 6 g

  Saturated 1 g

  Polyunsaturated 1 g

  Monounsaturated 3 g

Fiber 3 g

Sodium 28 mg

Mixed Fruit Salad with Mango Dressing

- Serves 8; ½ cup per serving
- Preparation time: 15 minutes

Experiment with different varieties of apple and with seasonal fruit when you make this refreshing salad.

1 large Fuji or Granny Smith apple
(about 8 ounces)

8 ounces fresh strawberries

3 small plums (2 to 3 ounces)

2 tablespoons dried cherries or other
dried fruit

1½ to 2 tablespoons fat-free mango
salad dressing, apricot or other
fruit nectar, or fat-free or light
raspberry vinaigrette salad dressing

½ cup alfalfa sprouts (1 ounce)
(optional)

Thinly slice apple, strawberries, and plums. Put in a medium bowl. Stir in cherries and salad dressing.

To serve, mound ½ cup fruit on each salad plate. Top each serving with 1 tablespoon alfalfa sprouts.

(PER SERVING)

Calories 36

Protein 1 g

Carbohydrates 9 g

Cholesterol 0 mg

Total Fat 0 g

  Saturated 0 g

  Polyunsaturated 0 g

  Monounsaturated 0 g

Fiber 1 g

Sodium 10 mg

Strawberry-Mango Salsa

Serves 6; ½ cup per serving ■
Preparation time: 20 minutes ■

This exciting, inviting salsa is especially delicious served with grilled pork or chicken.

1 fresh jalapeño

¼ cup lime juice (2 to 3 medium limes)

2 tablespoons sugar

1 teaspoon grated gingerroot

2 cups diced strawberries (about 1 pint)

1 medium mango, diced, or 1 cup diced refrigerated mango slices

1 to 2 tablespoons finely snipped fresh cilantro

Remove ribs and seeds from jalapeño; discard. Finely chop jalapeño.

In a medium bowl, whisk together lime juice, sugar, and gingerroot.

Stir in remaining ingredients, including jalapeño.

Serve immediately or cover and refrigerate for up to 1 hour. (Flavors are at their peak if served within 1 hour.)

PEACH SALSA

Replace strawberries with peaches, mango with blueberries or raspberries, lime juice with lemon juice, and cilantro with mint. Omit jalapeño. (Calories 67; Protein 1 g; Carbohydrates 17 g; Cholesterol 0 mg; Total Fat 0 g; Saturated 0 g; Polyunsaturated 0 g; Monounsaturated 0 g; Fiber 2 g; Sodium 4 mg)

COOK'S TIP ON HOT CHILE PEPPERS

Hot peppers, such as jalapeño, Anaheim, serrano, and poblano chile peppers, contain oils that can burn your skin, lips, and eyes. Wear rubber gloves or wash your hands thoroughly with warm, soapy water immediately after handling peppers.

(PER SERVING)

Calories 52

Protein 1 g

Carbohydrates 13 g

Cholesterol 0 mg

Total Fat 0 g

   Saturated 0 g

   Polyunsaturated 0 g

   Monounsaturated 0 g

Fiber 2 g

Sodium 2 mg

Orange-Pineapple Gelatin Salad

- Serves 8; ½ cup per serving
- Preparation time: 10 minutes
- Cooking time: 1 minute
- Chilling time: 4 hours

Buttermilk heightens the flavors of the fruit in this kid-pleasing salad or dessert.

8-ounce can crushed pineapple in its own juice

3-ounce package orange or mixed fruit gelatin (small package)

11-ounce can mandarin oranges in water or light syrup, well drained

1 cup fat-free or low-fat buttermilk

4 ounces frozen fat-free or light whipped topping, thawed (about 1½ cups)

8 lettuce leaves (optional)

2 cups Bing cherries or seedless red grapes (about 12 ounces of either) (optional)

In a small saucepan, bring undrained pineapple to a boil over high heat, about 1 minute. Remove from heat, add gelatin, and stir until gelatin is completely dissolved, about 1 minute. Pour into an 8- or 9-inch square glass baking dish and put in freezer for 5 to 8 minutes, or until beginning to set around edges.

Stir in oranges and buttermilk. Gently fold in whipped topping until well blended.

Chill, covered, until set, about 4 hours. Cut into 8 pieces and serve on lettuce with cherries.

(PER SERVING)

Calories 99

Protein 2 g

Carbohydrates 23 g

Cholesterol 1 mg

Total Fat 0 g

Saturated 0 g

Polyunsaturated 0 g

Monounsaturated 0 g

Fiber 1 g

Sodium 68 mg

LIME-PINEAPPLE GELATIN SALAD

Substitute lime or lemon gelatin for orange, nonfat or light sour cream for buttermilk, and fat-free or low-fat vanilla yogurt for whipped topping. (Calories 106; Protein 3 g; Carbohydrates 24 g; Cholesterol 3 mg; Total Fat 0 g; Saturated 0 g; Polyunsaturated 0 g; Monounsaturated 0 g; Fiber 1 g; Sodium 74 mg)

COOK'S TIP

Use sugar-free orange, lime, or lemon gelatin in place of regular to cut the calorie count.

German Potato Salad

Serves 6; ½ cup per serving ■
Preparation time: 10 minutes ■

Making potato salad is a great way to use leftover Roasted Red and White Potatoes. Whether you crave German or Mexican, we have a version for you.

3 cups Roasted Red and White Potatoes, room temperature or chilled (page 279)

¼ cup chopped celery

2 tablespoons cider vinegar

2 teaspoons snipped fresh dillweed

¼ teaspoon caraway seeds

2 tablespoons nonfat or light sour cream

1 tablespoon fat-free or light mayonnaise dressing

½ to 1 teaspoon hot German mustard

In a medium bowl, stir together potatoes, celery, vinegar, dillweed, and caraway seeds.

In a small bowl, whisk together remaining ingredients. Pour over potato mixture and stir well.

MEXICAN POTATO SALAD

3 cups Roasted Red and White Potatoes (page 279)

3 green onions, chopped (green and white parts) (about ⅓ cup)

2 tablespoons lime juice (1 to 2 medium limes)

2 teaspoons snipped fresh cilantro

2 teaspoons chopped canned jalapeños or green chiles, rinsed and drained (optional)

2 tablespoons fat-free or low-fat plain yogurt

2 tablespoons nonfat or light sour cream

In a medium bowl, stir together potatoes, green onions, lime juice, cilantro, and jalapeños.

In a small bowl, whisk together remaining ingredients. Pour over potato mixture and stir well. (Calories 105; Protein 3 g; Carbohydrates 22 g; Cholesterol 1 mg; Total Fat 1 g; Saturated 0 g; Polyunsaturated 0 g; Monounsaturated 1 g; Fiber 2 g; Sodium 78 mg)

(PER SERVING)

Calories 102

Protein 2 g

Carbohydrates 22 g

Cholesterol 1 mg

Total Fat 1 g

  Saturated 0 g

  Polyunsaturated 0 g

  Monounsaturated 1 g

Fiber 2 g

Sodium 102 mg

Barley and Vegetable Salad

- Serves 5; ½ cup per serving
- Preparation time: 10 minutes
- Cooking time: 10 to 12 minutes
- Standing time: 5 minutes
- Cooling time: 5 minutes

You can prepare this salad ahead and refrigerate it for up to four days, until you need a substantial side salad in a hurry. It looks so tempting you may not want to wait.

1½ cups water

½ cup uncooked quick-cooking barley

¼ teaspoon salt

2 ounces fresh asparagus

½ cup shredded red cabbage

¼ cup roasted red bell peppers, rinsed, drained, and chopped

1 green onion, thinly sliced

1 tablespoon feta cheese, rinsed and crumbled

2 teaspoons olive oil

2 teaspoons lemon juice

½ teaspoon dried oregano, crumbled

½ teaspoon sugar

In a medium saucepan, bring water to a boil over high heat. Stir in barley and salt; cook, covered, for 10 to 12 minutes, or until barley is tender.

Meanwhile, trim 1 inch from bottom of asparagus; discard trimmed portion. Cut spears into 1-inch pieces. Stir into cooked barley. Remove from heat and let stand, covered, for 5 minutes.

Drain any remaining liquid from barley mixture. Let mixture cool, uncovered, for 5 minutes.

In a large bowl, combine all ingredients.

Serve immediately or cover and chill.

(PER SERVING)

Calories 84

Protein 2 g

Carbohydrates 14 g

Cholesterol 2 mg

Total Fat 3 g

  Saturated 1 g

  Polyunsaturated 0 g

  Monounsaturated 1 g

Fiber 2 g

Sodium 202 mg

Italian Bean and Tuna Salad

Serves 3; 1 cup per serving ■
Preparation time: 10 minutes ■

Flavors of the Mediterranean blend in this simple, easy-to-love salad. Serve it as is or on lettuce.

15-ounce can cannellini or Great Northern beans, rinsed and drained

6-ounce can white tuna packed in spring or distilled water, rinsed and drained

¼ to ½ cup finely chopped red onion

3 tablespoons snipped fresh parsley or 1 tablespoon chopped fresh basil

2 to 3 tablespoons balsamic vinegar

1 tablespoon olive oil

¼ teaspoon freshly ground pepper

In a medium bowl, combine beans, tuna, onion, parsley, and vinegar.

Drizzle with oil, then sprinkle with pepper.

(PER SERVING)

Calories 221

Protein 20 g

Carbohydrates 24 g

Cholesterol 14 mg

Total Fat 5 g

  Saturated 1 g

  Polyunsaturated 1 g

  Monounsaturated 3 g

Fiber 7 g

Sodium 162 mg

Southwestern Chicken Salad

- Serves 6; 1 cup per serving
- Preparation time: 20 minutes
- Microwave time: 4 to 5 minutes *or*
  Cooking time: 17 minutes

Here's a new twist on chicken salad. Serve this one with fat-free tortilla chips on lettuce-lined plates, garnished with jalapeño rings.

Chicken Salad

4 boneless, skinless chicken breast halves (about 4 ounces each), all visible fat removed

½ medium red bell pepper

½ medium green bell pepper

¼ to ½ medium red onion

15-ounce can no-salt-added black beans, rinsed and drained

1 cup diced jícama

½ cup snipped fresh cilantro

½ fresh jalapeño, minced (optional)

Dressing

2 tablespoons olive oil

2 tablespoons orange juice

3 tablespoons cider vinegar

1 teaspoon ground cumin

½ teaspoon chili powder

½ teaspoon cayenne

½ teaspoon salt

Rinse chicken and pat dry with paper towels. Put chicken in a 9-inch microwave-safe pie plate and cover with wax paper. Microwave on 100 percent power (high) for 4 to 5 minutes, turning chicken halfway through cooking time. Or bring ½ inch water to a simmer in a large skillet and cook chicken, covered, for 15 minutes, or until barely pink in center. Set aside to finish cooking and cool.

Meanwhile, dice bell peppers and onion; put in a large bowl.

Add remaining chicken salad ingredients to bell pepper mixture, stirring well.

In a small jar with a tight-fitting lid, combine dressing ingredients. Shake to dissolve salt. Pour over bean mixture.

Chop chicken and add to bean mixture, tossing well. Serve immediately or cover and refrigerate until needed.

COOK'S TIP ON JÍCAMA

Jícama (HEE-kah-mah) is firm and barely sweet, like a fresh water chestnut. Its texture is somewhat applelike, but its flavor is much milder. A crunchy addition to raw vegetable platters, jícama is a refreshing dipper. Peel and slice or chop—that's it.

TIME-SAVER

Use 2 to 3 cups leftover cooked chicken or store-bought baked or rotisserie chicken instead of microwaving or poaching the chicken breast halves.

(PER SERVING)

Calories 215
Protein 22 g
Carbohydrates 15 g
Cholesterol 49 mg
Total Fat 7 g
  Saturated 1 g
  Polyunsaturated 1 g
  Monounsaturated 4 g
Fiber 4 g
Sodium 246 mg

Asian Chicken and Wild Rice Salad

- Serves 5; 1 cup per serving
- Preparation time: 10 minutes
- Cooking time: 8 minutes
- Cooling time: 8 minutes

If you can keep a secret, no one will guess that this delectable salad uses leftovers as a key ingredient.

7-ounce package quick-cooking white and wild rice

3 tablespoons light soy sauce

1 tablespoon plus 1½ teaspoons sugar

2 teaspoons rice vinegar

¼ teaspoon crushed red pepper flakes, or to taste

2 cups cooked Orange-Barbecue Chicken Chunks (page 150)

1 cup chopped red or green bell pepper (1 large)

8-ounce can sliced water chestnuts, rinsed, drained, and chopped

5 lettuce leaves (optional)

11-ounce can mandarin oranges in water or light syrup, drained (optional)

Cook rice using package directions, omitting salt, margarine, and seasoning packet.

Meanwhile, in a large bowl, whisk together soy sauce, sugar, vinegar, and red pepper flakes. Stir in chicken, bell pepper, and water chestnuts.

Spread cooked rice on a baking sheet in a thin layer. Put on a cooling rack and let stand for 8 minutes, or until rice has cooled, stirring occasionally. Stir into chicken mixture.

To serve, place a lettuce leaf on each plate and top with a mound of salad. Garnish with oranges.

COOK'S TIP ON RICE VINEGAR

When shopping for rice vinegar, read the nutrition label carefully. If it says "Seasoned Rice Vinegar," the product may have a lot of salt added. Mild and slightly sweet, pure rice vinegar has no sodium.

(PER SERVING)

Calories 335

Protein 25 g

Carbohydrates 53 g

Cholesterol 54 mg

Total Fat 3 g

  Saturated 1 g

  Polyunsaturated 1 g

  Monounsaturated 1 g

Fiber 3 g

Sodium 401 mg

Chicken and Grapefruit Salad

Serves 4; 3 cups per serving ■
Preparation time: 10 minutes ■
Cooking time: 8 minutes ■

A cooling, yet mildly spicy vinaigrette tops mixed salad greens, soy-brushed chicken, tangy grapefruit, and alfalfa sprouts.

Salad

4 boneless, skinless chicken breast halves (about 4 ounces each), all visible fat removed

Vegetable oil spray

1 tablespoon light soy sauce

8 cups mixed salad greens (about 8 ounces)

1 cup fresh grapefruit sections

½ cup thinly sliced red onion (about 2 ounces)

2 cups alfalfa sprouts (4 ounces)

Dressing

⅔ cup fresh grapefruit juice

1 tablespoon plus 1½ teaspoons honey

2 teaspoons cider vinegar

½ teaspoon crushed red pepper flakes

Rinse chicken and pat dry with paper towels.

Heat a large nonstick skillet over high heat until very hot. Remove from heat and spray with vegetable oil spray. Reduce heat to medium-high and cook chicken for 3 minutes. Brush tops with half the soy sauce, turn, and cook for 4 minutes, or until cooked through. Brush tops with remaining soy sauce and set aside on a plate to cool slightly.

Meanwhile, arrange 2 cups mixed salad greens on each of four plates. Top each with grapefruit and red onion. Place ½ cup alfalfa sprouts in center of each salad.

Cut chicken into thin strips and arrange on sprouts.

In a small bowl, whisk together dressing ingredients until well blended. Spoon over salads.

(PER SERVING)

Calories 222

Protein 29 g

Carbohydrates 19 g

Cholesterol 73 mg

Total Fat 3 g

  Saturated 1 g

  Polyunsaturated 1 g

  Monounsaturated 1 g

Fiber 2 g

Sodium 169 mg

Beef Salad with Vinaigrette Dressing

- Serves 4; 1 cup per serving
- Preparation time: 15 minutes

Here's an interesting lunch or light supper salad that uses cooked eye-of-round roast, such as leftovers from Tuscan Braised Beef (pages 196–197), and your choice of two dressings. You can even use leftovers of the leftovers tomorrow—any extra salad makes great sandwiches.

Beef Salad

3 ounces arugula or mixed baby greens

12 ounces cooked and chilled eye-of-round roast (about 12 thin slices)

⅛ teaspoon salt

Freshly ground pepper

½ small red onion, thinly sliced

1 teaspoon capers, rinsed and drained

Vinaigrette Dressing

3 tablespoons balsamic vinegar

¼ teaspoon Dijon mustard

¼ teaspoon bottled minced garlic

1 tablespoon extra-virgin olive oil

Stack arugula leaves on cutting board and cut crosswise at 1-inch intervals. Arrange on four salad plates.

Cut beef slices into ½ x 1-inch strips, about 3 cups. Arrange on arugula. Sprinkle with remaining salad ingredients.

For vinaigrette dressing, in a small bowl, whisk together vinegar, mustard, and garlic. Slowly whisk in oil.

To serve, top salad with dressing.

BEEF SALAD WITH HORSERADISH DRESSING

Prepare salad as above, substituting 4 medium radishes, thinly sliced, for red onion and capers. Instead of the vinaigrette dressing, whisk together ½ cup fat-free or low-fat plain yogurt; 1 tablespoon fat-free or light mayonnaise dressing; 1 teaspoon grated onion or onion juice, or to taste; and 1 to 1½ teaspoons prepared horseradish. Serves 4; 1 cup per serving. (Calories 173; Protein 27 g; Carbohydrates 4 g; Cholesterol 60 mg; Total Fat 5 g; Saturated 2 g; Polyunsaturated 0 g; Monounsaturated 2 g; Fiber 0 g; Sodium 190 mg)

COOK'S TIP ON BEEF YIELD

Beef shrinks about 25 percent when it cooks. To get 12 ounces of cooked meat, start with 1 pound.

(PER SERVING)

Calories 192
Protein 25 g
Carbohydrates 3 g
Cholesterol 59 mg
Total Fat 8 g
  Saturated 2 g
  Polyunsaturated 0 g
  Monounsaturated 5 g
Fiber 0 g
Sodium 145 mg

Thai Beef Salad

- Serves 4; 1 cup per serving
- Preparation time: 20 minutes

Turn leftover roast beef (such as Tuscan Braised Beef, pages 196–197) into a taste adventure by adding Thai-style dressing.

8 leaves of Boston lettuce

12 ounces cooked lean roast, cut into ½ x 1-inch strips

1 small cucumber, peeled and diced

½ small red onion, thinly sliced (about ½ cup)

Freshly ground pepper, to taste

Dressing

2 tablespoons lime juice (1 to 2 medium limes)

1 tablespoon sugar

1 tablespoon no-salt-added tomato paste

1 tablespoon fish sauce

1 tablespoon acceptable vegetable oil

1 teaspoon bottled minced garlic or 2 medium cloves garlic, minced

¼ teaspoon crushed red pepper flakes

■ ■ ■

1 tablespoon plus 1 teaspoon snipped fresh cilantro (optional)

Arrange 2 lettuce leaves on each of four salad plates. Put beef, cucumber, and onion in a medium bowl. Grind pepper over beef mixture and stir well.

For dressing, whisk together all ingredients in a small bowl. Stir into beef.

Arrange salad on lettuce and sprinkle with cilantro.

Cook's Tip on Fish Sauce

Thin and usually brown, fish sauce is a condiment made from salted, fermented fish, often anchovies. Its flavor and odor are pungent, so a little goes a long way. Thai fish sauce, *nam pla,* is milder than its Vietnamese counterpart, *nuoc mam.*

(PER SERVING)

Calories 210

Protein 26 g

Carbohydrates 7 g

Cholesterol 59 mg

Total Fat 9 g

　Saturated 2 g

　Polyunsaturated 2 g

　Monounsaturated 3 g

Fiber 1 g

Sodium 382 mg

Vegetarian Taco Salad

Serves 4; 3 cups per serving ■
Preparation time: 10 minutes ■

Such a simple meal, such a great taste. The fresh and tangy blend is wonderful by itself or with whatever additions you have on hand. Check your refrigerator for tomatoes, bell peppers, chiles, or corn to add to this flexible salad.

15-ounce can no-salt-added black beans, rinsed and drained, or 1 cup Mexican Bean Dip (page 38)

¼ to ½ cup salsa

8 cups chopped lettuce

8 ounces no-salt baked tortilla chips (about 2½ cups), slightly crushed

¾ to 1 cup shredded fat-free or reduced-fat Cheddar or Monterey Jack cheese (about 4 ounces)

¼ to ½ cup salsa

¼ cup fat-free or low-fat plain yogurt or nonfat or light sour cream (optional)

In a small bowl, combine beans with ¼ to ½ cup salsa. Mash slightly with a potato masher or fork.

To assemble, put 2 cups lettuce on each of four plates; sprinkle with chips. Spread bean mixture over each serving. Top with cheese, remaining salsa, and a dollop of yogurt.

(PER SERVING)

Calories 396

Protein 22 g

Carbohydrates 72 g

Cholesterol 2 mg

Total Fat 4 g

  Saturated 0 g

  Polyunsaturated —

  Monounsaturated —

Fiber 12 g

Sodium 416 mg

Fresh Herb Couscous Salad

- ■ Serves 8; 1½ cups per serving
- ■ Preparation time: 15 minutes
- ■ Cooling time: 15 minutes

The fresh herbs in this salad add an exotic flavor, similar to those found in Mediterranean dishes.

2 cups uncooked couscous

½ cup dried currants (optional)

½ teaspoon salt

3 cups boiling water

1 medium or large tomato

1 medium cucumber (about 8 ounces)

¼ to ½ cup chopped fresh mint or fresh cilantro

½ cup chopped mixed fresh herbs (such as chives, parsley, and basil)

¼ cup lemon juice (2 medium lemons)

¼ cup olive oil

½ teaspoon bottled minced garlic or 1 medium clove garlic, minced

Combine couscous, currants, and salt in a large bowl. Pour boiling water over mixture, stir to combine, and let cool for about 15 minutes.

Meanwhile, chop tomato; peel, seed, and chop cucumber. Add to cooled couscous with remaining ingredients and stir together.

Serve at room temperature or chilled.

(PER SERVING)

Calories 245

Protein 6 g

Carbohydrates 38 g

Cholesterol 0 mg

Total Fat 7 g

  Saturated 1 g

  Polyunsaturated 1 g

  Monounsaturated 5 g

Fiber 3 g

Sodium 159 mg

Orzo Salad with Green Peas and Artichokes

Serves 6; 1 cup per serving ■
Preparation time: 15 minutes ■
Cooking time: 15 minutes ■

This pleasant pasta salad is even tastier the second day. Enjoy it as an entrée or a side dish.

6 ounces uncooked orzo

1½ cups frozen green peas, thawed

⅓ cup finely chopped fresh basil or 2 tablespoons dried, crumbled

3 tablespoons cider vinegar

14.5-ounce can artichoke quarters, rinsed, drained, and cut in half lengthwise

7.2-ounce jar roasted red bell peppers, rinsed, drained, and chopped

2.5-ounce can sliced black olives, drained (½ cup)

¼ cup snipped fresh parsley (Italian, or flat-leaf, preferred) (optional)

2 teaspoons extra-virgin olive oil

⅛ teaspoon salt

Pepper to taste

Cook orzo using package directions, omitting salt and oil.

Meanwhile, in a large mixing bowl, stir together peas, basil, and vinegar. Stir in artichokes, roasted peppers, olives, and parsley.

Pour orzo into a colander and rinse under cold running water for 30 seconds to stop cooking process and cool quickly; drain well.

Stir orzo and remaining ingredients into artichoke mixture.

Serve immediately or cover with plastic wrap and refrigerate for up to 24 hours.

COOK'S TIP ON BOILING

To bring water to a boil quickly, start with hot tap water and cover the pot. If using an electric range, turn on the heat while running the tap water.

(PER SERVING)

Calories 161

Protein 6 g

Carbohydrates 29 g

Cholesterol 0 mg

Total Fat 3 g

  Saturated 0 g

  Polyunsaturated —

  Monounsaturated —

Fiber 4 g

Sodium 433 mg

Wheat Berry Salad

- Serves 5; ¼ cup per serving
- Preparation time: 20 minutes
- Cooking time: 50 minutes

While the wheat berries (whole kernels of wheat) cook, mix the rest of this unusual combination of ingredients. The resulting salad is crunchy, chewy, tangy, tart, and sweet—a texture and a flavor to suit everyone.

2 cups water

1 cup wheat berries (about 7 ounces)

10 ounces fresh cremini or button mushrooms

1 tablespoon acceptable vegetable oil

¼ teaspoon salt-free lemon pepper

¼ cup dried cherries or cranberries (about 1 ounce)

3 tablespoons sliced almonds

¼ cup maple syrup

2 tablespoons apple cider

1 tablespoon balsamic vinegar

2 tablespoons lime juice (1 to 2 medium limes)

Bring water to a boil in a large saucepan, covered, over high heat.

Meanwhile, rinse wheat berries. Add to boiling water and cook, covered, at a low boil for 45 minutes, or until water is nearly absorbed and wheat berries are crunchy-tender.

While wheat berries cook, quarter mushrooms.

Heat a large skillet over medium-high heat. Add oil and swirl to coat bottom of skillet. Add mushrooms and lemon pepper, stirring to coat. Cook, uncovered, for 7 to 10 minutes, or until just tender, stirring occasionally. Transfer mushrooms and juices to a large bowl.

Stir remaining ingredients except wheat berries into mushrooms.

Drain wheat berries and add to mushroom mixture, tossing well. Serve immediately or cover and refrigerate for up to three days.

(PER SERVING)

Calories 246

Protein 5 g

Carbohydrates 46 g

Cholesterol 0 mg

Total Fat 5 g

  Saturated 1 g

  Polyunsaturated 1 g

  Monounsaturated 3 g

Fiber 5 g

Sodium 7 mg

Far East Dressing

Serves 4; 1 tablespoon plus 1½ teaspoons per serving ■
Preparation time: 5 minutes ■

A little of this intensely flavored dressing goes a very long way. One tablespoon plus 1½ teaspoons is enough for about two cups of mixed salad greens.

3 tablespoons rice vinegar

2 tablespoons honey or dark brown sugar

2 teaspoons light soy sauce

2 teaspoons toasted sesame oil

¼ teaspoon crushed red pepper flakes, or to taste

In a small bowl, whisk together all ingredients until well blended.

Serve immediately or cover and refrigerate until needed.

FAR EAST CHICKEN SALAD

For a main-dish salad for one, add 3 ounces (about ½ cup) diced cooked skinless chicken breast to 2 cups mixed salad greens, 2 tablespoons thinly sliced red onion, and about half an 11-ounce can well-drained mandarin oranges (canned in water or light syrup, about ½ cup). Drizzle with 2 tablespoons Far East Dressing. (Calories 294; Protein 29 g; Carbohydrates 26 g; Cholesterol 72 mg; Total Fat 6 g; Saturated 1 g; Polyunsaturated 2 g; Monounsaturated 2 g; Fiber 4 g; Sodium 179 mg)

COOK'S TIP ON SESAME OIL

Be sure to use toasted sesame oil (also called Asian sesame oil) in this recipe because it has more flavor than regular sesame oil. Toasted sesame oil also is darker and more fragrant.

(PER SERVING)

Calories 55

Protein 0 g

Carbohydrates 9 g

Cholesterol 0 mg

Total Fat 2 g

  Saturated 0 g

  Polyunsaturated 1 g

  Monounsaturated 1 g

Fiber 0 g

Sodium 67 mg

Pepper Dijon Dressing

- Serves 8; 1 tablespoon per serving
- Preparation time: 5 minutes

Combine only five ingredients and get a simple blend that's just right with mixed salad greens, cucumbers, and artichoke hearts or with sliced tomatoes. This dressing is so full of flavor that you'll need only a tablespoon for a side salad.

¼ cup fat-free or low-fat plain yogurt

3 tablespoons Dijon mustard

2½ teaspoons lime juice or lemon juice

1½ teaspoons extra-virgin olive oil

1 teaspoon pepper

In a small bowl, whisk together all ingredients until well blended. Chill until needed.

TARRAGON DIJON DRESSING

For a more intensely flavored dressing, add 1 teaspoon finely chopped tarragon leaves or ¼ teaspoon dried tarragon, crumbled, with an additional 1 teaspoon lime juice. (Calories 18; Protein 0 g; Carbohydrates 2 g; Cholesterol 0 mg; Total Fat 1 g; Saturated 0 g; Polyunsaturated 0 g; Monounsaturated 1 g; Fiber 0 g; Sodium 140 mg)

COOK'S TIP

If you like your salad dressing a little thinner, add up to 1 tablespoon fat-free milk with the other ingredients.

(PER SERVING)

Calories 18

Protein 0 g

Carbohydrates 2 g

Cholesterol 0 mg

Total Fat 1 g

Saturated 0 g

Polyunsaturated 0 g

Monounsaturated 1 g

Fiber 0 g

Sodium 140 mg

Roasted Red Bell Pepper Dressing

Making this salad dressing is almost as effortless as opening bottled dressing, and you get the mellow taste of homemade. Serve over mixed salad greens with thinly sliced red onion, shredded cabbage, and snipped fresh cilantro.

7.2-ounce jar roasted red bell
  peppers, rinsed and drained

3 tablespoons balsamic vinegar

¼ teaspoon salt

1 tablespoon plus 1½ teaspoons extra-
  virgin olive oil

In a food processor or blender, process peppers, vinegar, and salt until smooth. Pour into a small bowl.

Stir oil into dressing.

Serve immediately or cover and chill until needed.

COOK'S TIP

For a thinner consistency, add 3 to 4 tablespoons water when you add the olive oil.

(PER SERVING)

Calories 30

Protein 0 g

Carbohydrates 2 g

Cholesterol 0 mg

Total Fat 3 g

  Saturated 0 g

  Polyunsaturated 0 g

  Monounsaturated 2 g

Fiber 0 g

Sodium 134 mg

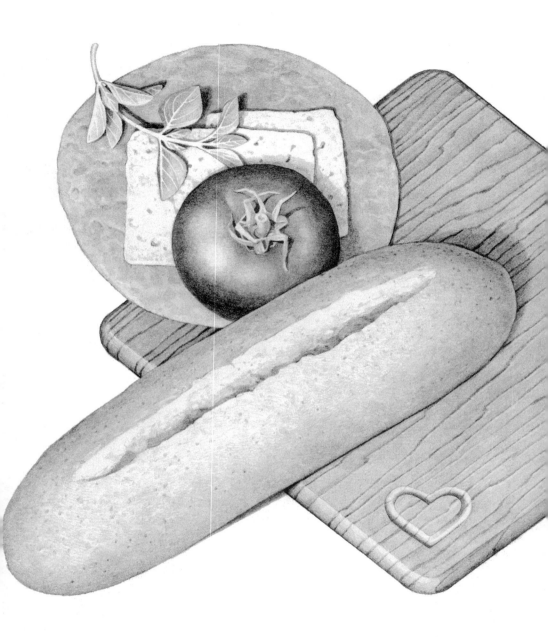

SANDWICHES

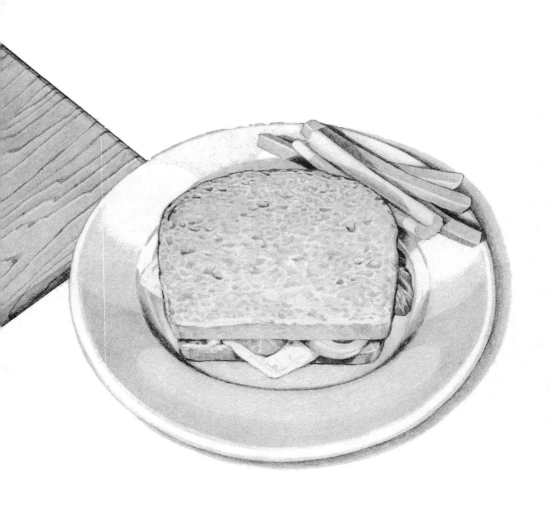

■ ■ ■

Tuna Pita Melts

Yucatecan Wraps

Barbecue Chicken Sloppy Joes

Cranberry and Cream Cheese
Turkey Sandwiches

Flank Steak Burritos

Beef and Caramelized Onion
on Hot French Bread

Tomato, Oregano, and Goat
Cheese Sandwiches

Portobello Sandwiches
with Zesty Red Onions

Open-Face Broiled Italian
Vegetable Sandwiches

Avocado Veggie Wraps

■ ■ ■

Tuna Pita Melts

Serves 4; 1 open-face sandwich per serving ■
Preparation time: 10 minutes ■
Cooking time: 10 minutes ■

Dress up tuna sandwiches by stacking the ingredients on toasted pita bread, then lightly toasting them. Serve the sandwiches with cucumber slices.

4 pita breads (leave whole)

6-ounce can albacore tuna packed in spring or distilled water, rinsed and drained

1 tablespoon fat-free or light mayonnaise dressing

1 tablespoon sweet pickle relish

¼ teaspoon dried dillweed, crumbled

⅛ teaspoon salt

1 medium tomato, cut into 12 wedges

¼ cup shredded fat-free or reduced-fat Cheddar cheese (about 1 ounce)

Preheat oven to 400° F.

Put pita breads in a single layer on a nonstick baking sheet. Bake for 5 minutes, or until lightly toasted.

Meanwhile, in a small bowl, combine tuna, salad dressing, pickle relish, dillweed, and salt.

To assemble, spread tuna mixture evenly on pita breads. Arrange tomato wedges on tuna. Sprinkle with Cheddar.

Bake for 5 minutes, or until cheese melts.

(PER SERVING)

Calories 232

Protein 17 g

Carbohydrates 36 g

Cholesterol 15 mg

Total Fat 2 g

　Saturated 0 g

　Polyunsaturated 0 g

　Monounsaturated 0 g

Fiber 3 g

Sodium 458 mg

Yucatecan Wraps

- Serves 4; 2 tortillas per serving
- Preparation time: 15 minutes
- Cooking time: 5 minutes

You can prepare dinner in a flash when you start with reserved Two-Way Border Chicken.

4 chicken breast halves and 1½ cups sauce reserved from Two-Way Border Chicken (page156)

2 tablespoons water

8 6-inch corn tortillas, warmed

½ cup finely chopped red onion

½ cup nonfat or light sour cream

¼ cup shredded fat-free or reduced-fat sharp Cheddar or Monterey Jack cheese (about 1 ounce)

¼ to ⅓ cup finely snipped fresh cilantro

Debone chicken and shred meat. Put meat, reserved sauce, and water in a medium saucepan; heat over medium-high heat for 4 to 5 minutes, or until thoroughly heated, stirring frequently. Remove from heat.

To assemble, spoon ¼ cup chicken mixture down center of each tortilla. Top with 1 tablespoon onion, 1 tablespoon sour cream, and 1½ teaspoons cheese. Sprinkle with cilantro. Roll tortilla jelly-roll style over filling and serve immediately.

(PER SERVING)

Calories 381

Protein 35 g

Carbohydrates 42 g

Cholesterol 77 mg

Total Fat 8 g

Saturated 2 g

Polyunsaturated 2 g

Monounsaturated 3 g

Fiber 5 g

Sodium 476 mg

COOK'S TIP ON WARMING TORTILLAS

To make tortillas (corn or flour) more pliable, warm them. Wrap the tortillas in aluminum foil and heat them in a 325° F or 350° F oven for 5 to 8 minutes. Another method is to wrap them in damp paper towels or put them in a tortilla warmer, then microwave them on 100 percent power (high) for 30 to 60 seconds. (Microwaving time depends on how many tortillas you're warming, as well as the wattage of your oven.)

Barbecue Chicken Sloppy Joes

Serves 4; 1 sandwich per serving ■

Preparation time: 10 minutes ■

Cooking time: 4 minutes ■

These sandwiches are indeed sloppy. In fact, you may want to eat them with a knife and fork. Buy a large enough chicken for the 2 cups you'll need here, with plenty to have leftovers. Then check the index for recipes that use cooked chicken, such as Sour Cream Chicken Enchiladas on page 170, or make more Sloppy Joes with the rest.

Barbecue Sauce

½ cup no-salt-added ketchup

⅓ cup water

2 tablespoons molasses

2 tablespoons cider vinegar

1 teaspoon Dijon mustard

■ ■ ■

½ cup canned sliced mushrooms, rinsed and drained

4 hamburger buns

2 cups rotisserie chicken, skin and all visible fat removed

In a medium saucepan, whisk together sauce ingredients. Cook over medium heat for about 1 minute.

Add mushrooms; reduce heat to medium-low and cook for about 3 minutes.

Meanwhile, to assemble, put one bun bottom on each of four plates. Put about ½ cup mixed white and dark meat on each.

Top with warm sauce and remaining bun pieces.

COOK'S TIP

For lighter eaters, use half a bun for each sandwich and serve open face.

(PER SERVING)

Calories 321

Protein 25 g

Carbohydrates 38 g

Cholesterol 62 mg

Total Fat 7 g

  Saturated 2 g

  Polyunsaturated 2 g

  Monounsaturated 3 g

Fiber 0 g

Sodium 345 mg

Cranberry and Cream Cheese Turkey Sandwiches

- Serves 4; ½ sandwich per serving
- Preparation time: 10 minutes

Holidays usually yield plenty of leftovers, which are handy for quick meals the next day. When you have extra turkey, use it to create this festive sandwich.

¼ cup fat-free or low-fat cream cheese, softened (2 ounces)

½ teaspoon grated orange zest

4 slices rye-pumpernickel swirl bread or 4 6-inch pita breads

8 ounces sliced skinless roasted turkey breast, all visible fat removed

4 curly endive leaves or red-tipped lettuce leaves

½ cup whole-berry cranberry sauce

In a small bowl, combine cream cheese and orange zest, stirring well.

Cut bread slices in half. Put four pieces on a cutting board or work surface.

To assemble, spread 1 tablespoon cream cheese mixture on each of the four bread slices. Top with turkey, endive, and cranberry sauce. Top with remaining bread.

COOK'S TIP ON PARTY SANDWICHES

For parties, assemble sandwiches as above, then cut each sandwich half crosswise into 3 pieces (you'll get 12 pieces). Arrange on a serving platter with large clusters of red and green grapes in the center.

(PER SERVING)

Calories 227

Protein 23 g

Carbohydrates 32 g

Cholesterol 50 mg

Total Fat 1 g

  Saturated 0 g

  Polyunsaturated 0 g

  Monounsaturated 0 g

Fiber 2 g

Sodium 330 mg

Flank Steak Burritos

Serves 4; 1 burrito per serving ■
Preparation time: 15 minutes ■
Microwave time: 3 minutes *or* ■
Cooking time: 5 minutes

You'll like these "pass arounds" because they use planned-overs from Taco-Rubbed Flank Steak. Your kids will like choosing their own combination of condiments and creating their own burritos. And everyone will like the taste.

2 cups shredded romaine or other lettuce

2 medium tomatoes, chopped

Chopped green onions (optional)

Nonfat or light sour cream (optional)

Salsa (optional)

Snipped fresh cilantro (optional)

6 ounces reserved meat from Taco-Rubbed Flank Steak (page 193), room temperature or heated briefly

½ cup cooked beans, such as pinto or kidney (no salt added if canned), mashed if desired

4 8-inch nonfat or low-fat flour tortillas

Put lettuce, tomatoes, green onions, sour cream, salsa, and cilantro in separate bowls.

Cut meat into ½-inch pieces; put in a serving dish.

Put beans in a small microwave-safe bowl. Microwave, covered, on 100 percent power (high) for 1 minute, or until hot, stirring once. Or warm in a small saucepan over medium-high heat for 1 to 2 minutes, stirring once.

Using package directions, heat tortillas in microwave or oven until soft and pliable.

To serve, let each diner fill and roll up (jelly-roll style) his or her own tortilla.

COOK'S TIP

For mashed beans with a slightly thinner consistency, warm them with several tablespoons of salsa or water. Start with 2 tablespoons, adding more if you wish.

(PER SERVING)

Calories 249

Protein 19 g

Carbohydrates 34 g

Cholesterol 27 mg

Total Fat 5 g

Saturated 2 g

Polyunsaturated 0 g

Monounsaturated 2 g

Fiber 4 g

Sodium 446 mg

Beef and Caramelized Onion on Hot French Bread

- Serves 4; 1 sandwich per serving
- Preparation time: 10 minutes
- Cooking time: 8 minutes

Now you can have sweet caramelized onion without a lot of time and effort. Cook the onion over high heat, add a bit of sugar, then reduce the heat to finish the process. If you planned ahead and have some Grilled Sirloin with Honey Mustard Marinade (page 187), it would be wonderful in this dish.

½ long, wide French bread (about 8 ounces)

Vegetable oil spray

1 large onion, thinly sliced (yellow preferred) (about 8 ounces)

1 teaspoon sugar

⅓ cup water

2 tablespoons fat-free or low-fat plain yogurt

1½ to 2 teaspoons prepared mustard

12 ounces reserved Grilled Sirloin with Honey Mustard Marinade or other cooked lean beef, thinly sliced

Preheat oven to 300° F. Wrap bread in aluminum foil and put in oven.

Heat a large nonstick skillet over high heat. Remove skillet from heat and spray with vegetable oil spray. Cook onion for 3 minutes, stirring constantly. Reduce heat to medium-high.

Add sugar and cook for 3 minutes, or until onion is richly browned, stirring constantly. Stir in water. Remove skillet from heat.

In a small bowl, whisk together yogurt and mustard until completely blended.

Cut bread in half lengthwise, then cut each half crosswise into fourths (eight pieces). Spread yogurt mixture on cut side of four pieces; top with beef, then with onion and remaining bread slices.

(PER SERVING)

Calories 368

Protein 28 g

Carbohydrates 40 g

Cholesterol 65 mg

Total Fat 8 g

Saturated 3 g

Polyunsaturated 0 g

Monounsaturated 2 g

Fiber 3 g

Sodium 473 mg

Tomato, Oregano, and Goat Cheese Sandwiches

Serves 4; 2 open-face sandwiches per serving ■
Preparation time: 10 minutes ■

This simple sandwich is simply terrific. It's best when tomatoes are in full flavor and color.

4 ounces goat cheese, softened

8 slices peasant or sourdough bread, about 1 inch thick (1 ounce per slice)

2 large tomatoes

2 sprigs of fresh oregano

Freshly ground pepper

Balsamic vinegar

Scant ¼ teaspoon extra-virgin olive oil (optional)

Slice cheese into eight pieces and spread on bread.

Remove and discard seeds from tomatoes, then cut tomatoes into ¼-inch slices.

To assemble, put tomatoes on cheese. Sprinkle with oregano leaves. Grind pepper over each sandwich and drizzle sparingly with vinegar. Top each sandwich with about 3 drops olive oil.

COOK'S TIP

If the loaf of bread is large, use four slices. Cut each one in half for easier eating.

(PER SERVING)

Calories 249

Protein 11 g

Carbohydrates 34 g

Cholesterol 13 mg

Total Fat 8 g

  Saturated 5 g

  Polyunsaturated 1 g

  Monounsaturated 2 g

Fiber 3 g

Sodium 459 mg

Portobello Sandwiches with Zesty Red Onions

- Serves 4; 1 sandwich per serving
- Preparation time: 15 minutes
- Cooking time: 18 to 20 minutes

Layers of mushroom slices, red bell peppers, and cheese, all seasoned with a sweet-and-sour onion mixture, combine to create a unique sandwich.

Vegetable oil spray

3 tablespoons low-sodium vegetable broth, low-sodium chicken broth, or water

1 teaspoon toasted sesame oil

2 small or medium red onions, sliced ¼ inch thick (1 to 2 cups)

1 large or 2 medium red bell peppers, sliced

2 tablespoons light brown sugar

1 tablespoon vinegar

1 tablespoon lemon juice

1 teaspoon dried basil, crushed, or 1 tablespoon snipped fresh basil

⅛ to ¼ teaspoon crushed red pepper flakes

2 fresh portobello mushrooms (6 to 8 ounces), stems discarded

½ long, wide loaf French or Italian bread (about ½ pound)

2 ounces provolone cheese, sliced

Spray a large nonstick skillet, roasting pan, and roasting rack with vegetable oil spray.

Pour broth and oil into skillet; swirl to coat bottom. Cook onions and peppers over medium-high heat for 2 minutes, stirring occasionally. Reduce heat to medium and cook until onions are quite limp and beginning to brown, about 10 minutes, stirring occasionally.

Meanwhile, preheat broiler.

In a small bowl, whisk together brown sugar, vinegar, lemon juice, basil, and red pepper flakes until sugar dissolves. Lightly brush both sides of mushrooms with mixture.

Broil mushrooms on roasting rack about 4 inches from heat for 5 minutes on each side, or until they darken and begin to shrivel.

When onions are beginning to brown, stir in remaining brown sugar mixture. Boil over medium heat until onions are coated and no liquid remains.

Slice bread in half lengthwise, then in quarters cross-wise (8 pieces); cut mushrooms into ¼-inch slices.

To assemble, spread onion mixture over four pieces of bread. Add mushrooms, then provolone. Top with remaining bread and serve. Or put open sandwiches and remaining bread on the roasting rack used for mushrooms and broil for 1 minute, or until cheese melts and bread is toasted.

Cook's Tip

You can use half as much bread as the recipe calls for and serve this sandwich open-face. You'll need knives and forks.

(PER SERVING)

Calories 306

Protein 12 g

Carbohydrates 49 g

Cholesterol 12 mg

Total Fat 7 g

   Saturated 3 g

    Polyunsaturated 1 g

    Monounsaturated 2 g

Fiber 3 g

Sodium 463 mg

Open-Face Broiled Italian Vegetable Sandwiches

- Serves 4; 1 open-face sandwich per serving
- Preparation time: 10 minutes
- Cooking time: 8 minutes

Basil-infused vinaigrette coats the bread as well as the veggies that are stacked high for these colorful sandwiches.

Vegetable oil spray

1 small eggplant, cut lengthwise into 4 slices (about 12 ounces)

1 large zucchini, cut lengthwise into ¼-inch slices (about 7 ounces)

1 large crookneck squash, cut cross-wise into ¼-inch slices (about 7 ounces)

½ long, wide loaf French bread (about 8 ounces)

Vinaigrette

2 tablespoons finely chopped fresh basil or 2 teaspoons dried, crumbled

1 tablespoon plus 1½ teaspoons red wine vinegar

1 tablespoon extra-virgin olive oil

½ teaspoon bottled minced garlic or 1 medium garlic clove, minced

⅛ teaspoon salt

■ ■ ■

1 extra-large tomato, cut into 8 slices (about 8 ounces)

(PER SERVING)

Calories 244
Protein 7 g
Carbohydrates 43 g
Cholesterol 2 mg
Total Fat 6 g
  Saturated 1 g
  Polyunsaturated 1 g
  Monounsaturated 3 g
Fiber 5 g
Sodium 415 mg

Preheat broiler.

Line a baking sheet with aluminum foil. Spray foil with vegetable oil spray. Arrange eggplant, zucchini, and crookneck squash in a single layer on baking sheet. Lightly spray tops with vegetable oil spray.

Broil vegetables about 4 inches from heat for 4 minutes, or until lightly brown. Turn vegetables over and lightly spray with vegetable oil spray. Broil for 4 minutes, or until lightly brown.

Meanwhile, cut bread in half lengthwise, then in half crosswise (4 pieces). In a small bowl, whisk together vinaigrette ingredients. Using a pastry brush, brush half the vinaigrette over cut side of bread.

Arrange tomato slices on bread, then top with broiled vegetables. Brush with remaining vinaigrette.

Avocado Veggie Wraps

Serves 4; 1 sandwich per serving ■
Preparation time: 15 minutes ■
Warming time: 10 minutes *or* ■
Microwave time: 20 to 30 seconds

Bulging with crispy vegetables, this California-style pita wrap is topped with a lime and sour cream dressing.

4 6-inch plain pita rounds

1 cup canned no-salt-added chick-peas, rinsed and drained

1 cup diced cucumber

1 medium tomato, seeded and chopped (5 to 6 ounces)

1 medium avocado, diced (about 1 cup)

¼ cup finely chopped red onion

½ cup nonfat or light sour cream

2 tablespoons fat-free milk

1 tablespoon plus 1½ teaspoons lime juice

¼ teaspoon salt

1 cup alfalfa sprouts (2 ounces)

Preheat oven to 350° F. Wrap pita rounds in aluminum foil and heat for 10 minutes, or until warmed through. Or put pita rounds on a microwave-safe plate and cover with plastic wrap or damp paper towels. Microwave on 100 percent power (high) for 20 to 30 seconds, or until warmed through.

Meanwhile, in a large bowl, combine chick-peas, cucumber, tomato, avocado, and onion; set aside.

In a small bowl, whisk together sour cream, milk, lime juice, and salt until smooth. Add to chick-pea mixture and stir gently.

To assemble, place one fourth of mixture and one fourth of alfalfa sprouts down center of each pita. Roll up jelly-roll style and secure each wrap by inserting two 6-inch bamboo skewers in an X through the pita.

(PER SERVING)

Calories 285

Protein 10 g

Carbohydrates 42 g

Cholesterol 3 mg

Total Fat 10 g

   Saturated 1 g

   Polyunsaturated 2 g

   Monounsaturated 5 g

Fiber 9 g

Sodium 371 mg

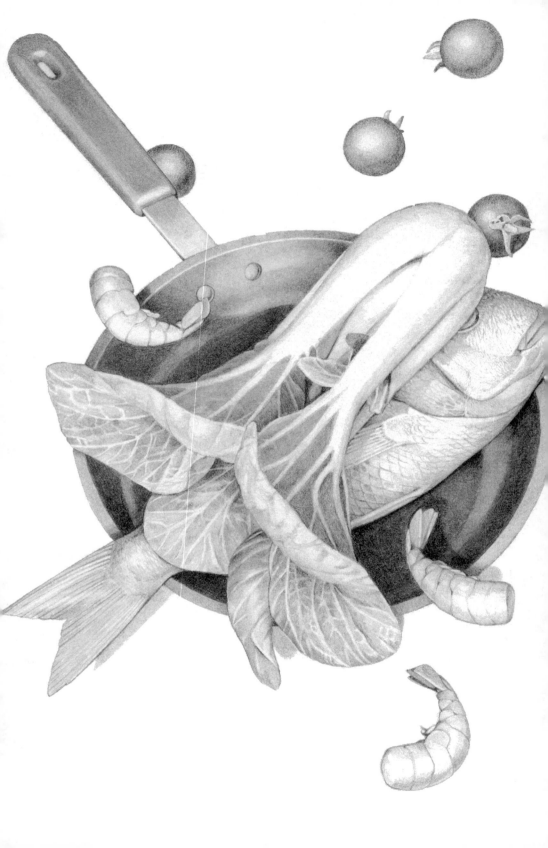

SEAFOOD

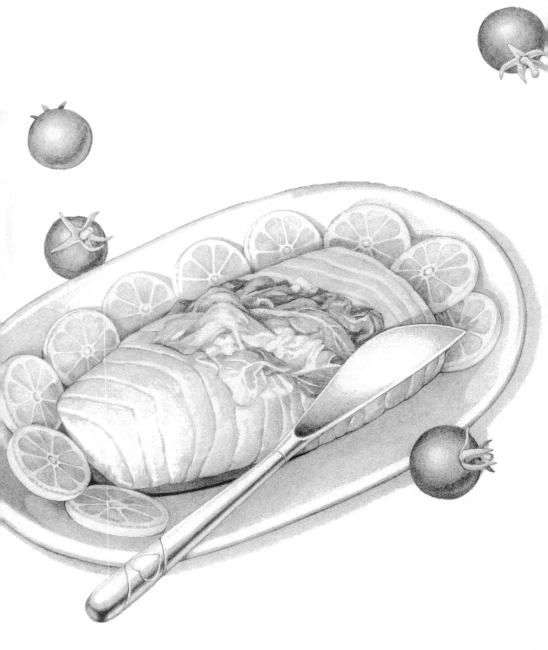

■ ■ ■

Halibut and Vegetable Medley

Orange Roughy with Bok Choy
and Cherry Tomatoes

Salmon Sorrento

Honey Mustard Salmon

Broiled Salmon-Stuffed
Tomatoes

Scrod Veracruz

Portuguese Sea Bass

Citrus Sole

Sole and Vegetable Terrine

Sole Mozzarella

Tilapia with Artichokes
and Sun-Dried Tomatoes

Grilled Tuna with Garlic

Hawaiian-Style Tuna

Grilled Tuna Niçoise

Tuna Casserole with Broccoli
and Water Chestnuts

Penne Pasta with Tuna
Marinara Sauce

Fish Bundles

Crumb-Crusted Fish Fillets

   Cajun Baked Fish

Fish with Chunky Creole Sauce

Scallops Provençal

Pan-Blackened Scallops
over Lemon Rice

Barbecue Shrimp Kebabs

Shrimp Marsala

Spanish Shrimp

Mixed Kebabs

   Italian Marinade

   Tex-Mex Marinade

   Asian Marinade

■ ■ ■

Halibut and Vegetable N

Serves 4; 1 cup per serving ▬

Preparation time: 5 minutes ■

Cooking time: 18 to 19 minutes ■

Mixed Fruit Salad with Mango Dressing (page 76) and rolls are all you need to complete the meal when you serve this easy dish.

12 ounces halibut, tuna, or shark

2 teaspoons olive oil

1 teaspoon bottled minced garlic or 2 medium cloves garlic, chopped

20-ounce bag mixed frozen vegetables (stew vegetables preferred)

½ teaspoon seafood or fish seasoning

⅛ teaspoon cayenne

⅛ teaspoon salt

Freshly ground pepper to taste

Rinse fish and pat dry with paper towels. Cut fish into 2-inch pieces.

Heat a large skillet over medium heat. Add olive oil and swirl to coat bottom of skillet. Cook garlic until golden brown, 1 to 2 minutes.

Add remaining ingredients except halibut. Cook, covered, for 10 minutes.

Add halibut and cook, covered, for 6 minutes, or until fish flakes easily when tested with a fork and ingredients are heated through, stirring occasionally.

(PER SERVING)

Calories 222

Protein 23 g

Carbohydrates 23 g

Cholesterol 27 mg

Total Fat 5 g

   Saturated 1 g

    Polyunsaturated 1 g

    Monounsaturated 2 g

Fiber 8 g

Sodium 276 mg

Orange Roughy with Bok Choy and Cherry Tomatoes

- Serves 4; 3 ounces fish and ¼ cup sauce per serving
- Preparation time: 15 minutes
- Cooking time: 17 to 20 minutes

Bok choy is traditionally used in stir-fry dishes, but rules can be broken! This recipe incorporates the crispy white stalks and spinachlike leaves into a creamy sauce that's accented with cherry tomatoes and served over poached fish.

1 teaspoon light margarine

½ medium onion, thinly sliced

1 pound orange roughy, cod, tilapia, or red snapper fillets

½ cup low-sodium chicken broth

½ cup dry white wine (regular or nonalcoholic)

⅛ teaspoon pepper

1 cup cherry tomatoes (about ½ pint)

1 small bunch bok choy (12 ounces to 1 pound)

3 tablespoons water

1 tablespoon plus 1½ teaspoons all-purpose flour

¼ cup nonfat or light sour cream, room temperature

Heat a large skillet over medium-high heat. Add margarine and onions and cook for 2 to 3 minutes, or until onions are translucent, stirring occasionally.

Rinse fish and pat dry with paper towels. Add fish, broth, wine, and pepper to skillet; bring to a simmer over medium-high heat. Reduce heat to low and cook, covered, for 8 to 10 minutes, or until fish flakes easily when tested with a fork.

Meanwhile, slice cherry tomatoes in half and put them in a medium bowl; set aside.

Trim and discard ends of bok choy stalks. Slice stalks into ¼-inch pieces. Cut bok choy leaves into thin strips and set aside.

In a small bowl, whisk together water and flour; set aside.

When fish is done, transfer to a serving platter, using a slotted spoon. Cover with aluminum foil to keep warm. (Fish will continue to cook slightly as it sits.)

Add bok choy to skillet; bring to a simmer over

medium-high heat. Cook for 1 to 2 minutes, or until tender-crisp, stirring occasionally.

Stir in flour mixture and cook over medium-high heat for 1 to 2 minutes, or until thick and bubbly, stirring occasionally. Reduce heat to low.

Add bok choy leaves and tomatoes; cook for 1 to 2 minutes, or until leaves are tender and mixture cools slightly, stirring occasionally. Remove from heat.

Stir in sour cream. Cook over low heat for 1 to 2 minutes, or until warmed through, stirring occasionally. Spoon over fish.

COOK'S TIP ON BOK CHOY

To make slicing bok choy easier, stack the leaves and roll them up together, starting from a long side. Slice the roll crosswise into thin strips.

(PER SERVING)

Calories 153

Protein 20 g

Carbohydrates 10 g

Cholesterol 25 mg

Total Fat 1 g

  Saturated 0 g

  Polyunsaturated 0 g

  Monounsaturated 1 g

Fiber 2 g

Sodium 168 mg

Salmon Sorrento

- Serves 4; 3 ounces fish per serving
- Preparation time: 10 minutes
- Cooking time: 23 to 26 minutes

With its thick, colorful sauce, this dish provides a way to dress up salmon without covering up its natural flavor.

1 tablespoon extra-virgin olive oil

5 medium Italian plum tomatoes, diced

6 medium black olives, coarsely chopped

6 medium green olives, coarsely chopped

3 tablespoons lemon juice

2 tablespoons coarsely or finely chopped fresh parsley (Italian, or flat-leaf, preferred)

1 tablespoon capers, rinsed and drained

1½ teaspoons bottled minced garlic or 3 medium cloves garlic, thinly sliced

Pepper to taste

1-pound salmon fillet

Heat a large skillet over medium-high heat. Add oil and swirl to coat bottom of skillet. Add tomatoes, black and green olives, lemon juice, parsley, capers, garlic, and pepper; stir to mix. Bring to a boil over medium-high heat, 2 to 3 minutes. Reduce heat to medium and cook until mixture is reduced by about one third, about 5 minutes, stirring occasionally.

Meanwhile, rinse salmon and pat dry with paper towels.

Using a spoon, push reduced sauce to one side and place salmon in skillet. Spoon sauce over salmon. Cook, covered, over medium heat for 15 to 17 minutes, or until salmon flakes easily when tested with a fork.

(PER SERVING)

Calories 202

Protein 24 g

Carbohydrates 6 g

Cholesterol 84 mg

Total Fat 9 g

   Saturated 2 g

   Polyunsaturated 1 g

   Monounsaturated 5 g

Fiber 1 g

Sodium 337 mg

Honey Mustard Salmon

Serves 6; 3 ounces fish per serving ■
Preparation time: 5 minutes ■
Cooking time: 6 minutes ■

This dish is elegant enough for company, quick enough for a "desperation dinner," and convenient enough for any cook. You can put it together at the last minute or assemble it in the morning so it's ready to cook when you are.

2 tablespoons snipped fresh dillweed or 1 teaspoon dried, crumbled

2 tablespoons Dijon mustard or any other good-quality mustard

1 tablespoon honey

6 salmon fillets (about 4 ounces each)

Vegetable oil spray (optional)

Preheat grill on high or preheat broiler to 450° F.

In a small bowl, whisk together dillweed, mustard, and honey.

Rinse salmon and pat dry with paper towels. Brush mustard mixture all over flesh side of salmon.

If broiling fish, spray a baking sheet with vegetable oil spray. Put fish skin side down on grill or baking sheet. Grill or broil about 6 inches from heat for about 6 minutes, or until fish is barely translucent at its thickest part and sides are beginning to flake when tested with a fork. Fish will cook a little more after you remove it from the heat.

(PER SERVING)

Calories 152

Protein 23 g

Carbohydrates 4 g

Cholesterol 84 mg

Total Fat 4 g

Saturated 1 g

Polyunsaturated 1 g

Monounsaturated 2 g

Fiber 0 g

Sodium 177 mg

Broiled Salmon-Stuffed Tomatoes

- Serves 4; 1 stuffed tomato per serving
- Preparation time: 5 minutes
- Cooking time: 10 minutes

Complement this easy dish with crunchy baby carrots and strips of cucumber and bell pepper.

7½-ounce can salmon, skin removed, drained

½ cup plain dry bread crumbs

¼ cup frozen green peas

3 tablespoons Dijon mustard

2 tablespoons snipped fresh parsley

4 large tomatoes (about 8 ounces each)

Preheat broiler.

In a medium bowl, combine all ingredients except tomatoes, stirring well.

Core tomatoes, leaving a ¼- to ½-inch shell; discard pulp. Stuff tomatoes and place in a small, shallow broilerproof pan.

Broil 5 to 6 inches from heat for 4 to 5 minutes. Move to lowest rack and broil for 5 minutes.

Cook's Tip on Coring and Seeding Tomatoes

Cut about ½ inch from the top of the tomatoes. With a grapefruit spoon or other small metal spoon, scoop out the pulp and seeds. If you don't need the tomatoes to retain their shape, you can instead cut them crosswise and squeeze out the seeds and liquid.

(PER SERVING)

Calories 165

Protein 13 g

Carbohydrates 21 g

Cholesterol 17 mg

Total Fat 4 g

Saturated 1 g

Polyunsaturated 1 g

Monounsaturated 1 g

Fiber 3 g

Sodium 444 mg

Scrod Veracruz

Serves 4; 3 ounces fish per serving ■
Preparation time: 5 minutes ■
Cooking time: 15 to 20 minutes ■

Some like it hot, so here's the perfect spicy fish dish. While it bakes, you'll have time to prepare corn on the cob and steamed zucchini.

Vegetable oil spray

1 pound scrod, grouper, snapper, orange roughy, or other white fish fillets

½ cup salsa

2 tablespoons plain dry bread crumbs

2 tablespoons shredded reduced-fat Monterey Jack or fat-free or reduced-fat mozzarella cheese

Preheat oven to 375° F. Spray a 12 x 8 x 2-inch baking pan with vegetable oil spray.

Rinse fish and pat dry with paper towels. Put fish in pan and top with salsa, bread crumbs, and cheese.

Bake for 15 to 20 minutes, or until fish flakes easily when tested with a fork.

(PER SERVING)

Calories 130

Protein 22 g

Carbohydrates 5 g

Cholesterol 50 mg

Total Fat 2 g

   Saturated 1 g

   Polyunsaturated 0 g

   Monounsaturated 0 g

Fiber 1 g

Sodium 221 mg

Portuguese Sea Bass

- Serves 4; 3 ounces fish per serving
- Preparation time: 10 minutes
- Cooking time: 20 minutes

Green spinach and red tomato contrast handsomely with white-flesh fish in this dish. Microwave potatoes to round out the meal.

Vegetable oil spray (olive oil spray preferred)

1 pound sea bass, cod, orange roughy, sole, or any other white fish fillets

10-ounce package frozen chopped spinach, thawed

¼ teaspoon salt

Pepper to taste

1 medium tomato, thinly sliced

1 small onion, sliced into thin rings (about ½ cup)

1 tablespoon olive oil

1 tablespoon red wine vinegar

1 tablespoon lemon juice

Preheat oven to 400° F. Spray an 11 x 7 x 1½-inch baking pan with vegetable oil spray. Rinse fish and pat dry with paper towels.

To assemble, spread spinach in pan; place fish on spinach. Sprinkle with salt and pepper, then top with tomato and onion. Drizzle with olive oil, vinegar, and lemon juice.

Bake, uncovered, for 20 minutes, or until fish flakes easily when tested with a fork.

(PER SERVING)

Calories 173

Protein 24 g

Carbohydrates 8 g

Cholesterol 47 mg

Total Fat 6 g

  Saturated 1 g

  Polyunsaturated 1 g

  Monounsaturated 3 g

Fiber 3 g

Sodium 285 mg

Citrus Sole

Serves 4; 3 ounces fish per serving ■
Preparation time: 5 minutes ■
Cooking time: 18 to 20 minutes ■

Orange marmalade brings a completely different taste to an already wonderful combination of citrus and seafood.

Vegetable oil spray

1 pound sole, scrod, or orange roughy fillets

2 tablespoons lemon juice

2 tablespoons lime juice (1 to 2 medium limes)

1 to 1 tablespoon plus 1½ teaspoons all-fruit orange marmalade

Preheat oven to 375° F. Spray a 12 x 8 x 2-inch baking pan with vegetable oil spray.

Rinse fish and pat dry with paper towels.

In a small bowl, stir together remaining ingredients. Using a basting brush, coat both sides of fish. Put fish in pan.

Bake for 18 to 20 minutes, or until fish flakes easily when tested with a fork.

(PER SERVING)

Calories 121

Protein 21 g

Carbohydrates 5 g

Cholesterol 60 mg

Total Fat 1 g

  Saturated 0 g

  Polyunsaturated 0 g

  Monounsaturated 0 g

Fiber 0 g

Sodium 98 mg

Sole and Vegetable Terrine

- Serves 4; 1 slice per serving
- Preparation time: 10 minutes
- Cooking time: 43 to 49 minutes *or*
  Microwave time: 13 to 15 minutes

This seafood loaf alternates layers of thin sole fillets with colorful carrots, tomato, and zucchini. Serve with steamed red potatoes and Peach Fans on Blackberry-Lime Sauce (page 74).

Olive oil spray

1 pound sole fillets

1 teaspoon olive oil

2 medium leeks, cut into thin strips (white part only) (about 1 cup)

1 medium carrot, cut into thin strips

1 teaspoon bottled minced garlic or 2 medium cloves garlic, minced

1 teaspoon herbes de Provence or salt-free herb combination

¼ teaspoon salt

⅛ teaspoon pepper

1 medium zucchini, thinly sliced

2 medium Italian plum tomatoes, thinly sliced

½ cup low-sodium chicken broth

Preheat oven to 425° F. Spray an 8½ x 4½ x 2½-inch loaf pan with olive oil spray. Line pan with parchment paper (optional).

Rinse sole and pat dry with paper towels. Cut sole into nine pieces; set aside.

Heat a medium skillet over medium heat. Add olive oil and swirl to coat bottom of skillet. Cook leeks, carrot, and garlic for 2 to 3 minutes, or until vegetables are tender, stirring occasionally.

In a small bowl, stir together herbes de Provence, salt, and pepper.

To assemble terrine, place three pieces of sole in loaf pan. Arrange one third of leek mixture over sole. Top with one third of zucchini and tomatoes. Sprinkle with one third of herb mixture. Repeat layers twice. Pour broth over all. Cover pan tightly with aluminum foil.

Bake for 40 to 45 minutes, or until fish flakes easily when tested with a fork. (The internal temperature of the mixture should read 137° F to 145° F on an instant-read thermometer.)

Uncover pan and lift up on parchment paper, letting liquid drain into pan; remove terrine from pan. (If you aren't using parchment paper, drain liquid and invert pan or use a spatula.) Cut terrine into four slices.

MICROWAVE METHOD

Spray an 8½ x 4½ x 2½-inch microwave-safe glass loaf pan with olive oil spray (line with parchment paper if desired). Assemble terrine as directed above (no need to cook leek mixture). Cover pan tightly with plastic wrap. Cook on 100 percent power (high) for 13 to 15 minutes, or until the internal temperature reads 137° F to 145° F on an instant-read thermometer.

COOK'S TIP ON HERBES DE PROVENCE

A blend of flavors favored in French cooking, herbes de Provence is available in the spice section of the grocery store. If you don't find it, you can make your own mixture of equal amounts of two or more of the following dried herbs: basil, rosemary, sage, thyme, and lavender.

(PER SERVING)

Calories 176

Protein 24 g

Carbohydrates 13 g

Cholesterol 60 mg

Total Fat 3 g

  Saturated 1 g

  Polyunsaturated 1 g

  Monounsaturated 1 g

Fiber 2 g

Sodium 276 mg

Sole Mozzarella

- Serves 4; 3 ounces fish per serving
- Preparation time: 15 minutes
- Cooking time: 9 minutes

To prepare this Italian specialty with a fraction of the usual fat and cholesterol, just use egg substitute and nonfat or part-skim mozzarella cheese. It's as simple as that.

Egg substitute equivalent to 3 eggs

¾ cup plain dry bread crumbs

1 pound white fish fillets, such as sole, perch, scrod, orange roughy, or tilapia

Vegetable oil spray

1½ cups canned no-salt-added tomato sauce (12 ounces)

½ teaspoon bottled minced garlic or 1 medium clove garlic, minced

¼ teaspoon salt-free Italian seasoning, crumbled

⅓ cup nonfat or part-skim mozzarella cheese

1 tablespoon snipped fresh parsley (Italian, or flat-leaf, preferred)

Pour egg substitute into a shallow medium bowl. Put bread crumbs on a plate. Cut a piece of wax paper about 12 inches long. Set bowl, plate, and wax paper in a row.

Rinse fish and pat dry with paper towels.

Spray a large skillet with vegetable oil spray. Put over medium heat.

Dip one piece of fish into egg mixture, turning to coat. Repeat with bread crumbs. Put on wax paper. Repeat with remaining fillets. Arrange fish in skillet. Cook for 3 minutes; turn and cook for 2 minutes. Reduce heat to low.

Combine tomato sauce, garlic, and Italian seasoning; pour over fish. Cook, covered, for 2 minutes.

Sprinkle with mozzarella and cook, covered, for 2 minutes, or until fish flakes easily when tested with a fork.

To serve, sprinkle with parsley.

(PER SERVING)

Calories 249

Protein 32 g

Carbohydrates 22 g

Cholesterol 62 mg

Total Fat 3 g

  Saturated 1 g

  Polyunsaturated 1 g

  Monounsaturated 1 g

Fiber 2 g

Sodium 459 mg

Tilapia with Artichokes and Sun-Dried Tomatoes

Serves 4; 3 ounces fish per serving ■
Preparation time: 10 minutes ■
Cooking time: 8 minutes ■

Tilapia, a farm-raised fish, has a very delicate flavor, similar to that of sole. In this recipe, tilapia combines superbly with white wine, sun-dried tomatoes, and artichoke hearts for a dish fit for almost any occasion.

4 tilapia or sole fillets (about 4 ounces each)

1 tablespoon all-purpose flour

2 tablespoons extra-virgin olive oil

1 teaspoon bottled chopped garlic or 2 medium cloves garlic, chopped

½ cup dry white wine (regular or nonalcoholic)

½ cup fat-free evaporated milk

¼ cup plus 2 tablespoons lemon juice (2 medium lemons)

½ 9-ounce package frozen artichoke hearts or ½ 14-ounce can artichokes, quartered (rinsed and drained if canned)

2 sun-dried tomatoes, dry packed (4 halves), chopped

Pepper to taste

Rinse fish and pat dry with paper towels. Sprinkle flour on both sides of fish. Heat a large skillet over medium heat. Add oil and swirl to coat bottom of skillet. Cook fish for 3 minutes. Turn fish over and cook for 2 minutes; sprinkle with garlic and cook for 1 minute.

Increase heat to high and add remaining ingredients. Cook for 6 to 8 minutes, or until sauce thickens to desired consistency, stirring occasionally.

(PER SERVING)

Calories 238

Protein 26 g

Carbohydrates 13 g

Cholesterol 61 mg

Total Fat 9 g

   Saturated 1 g

    Polyunsaturated 1 g

    Monounsaturated 5 g

Fiber 2 g

Sodium 226 mg

Grilled Tuna with Garlic

- Serves 4; 3 ounces fish per serving
- Preparation time: 10 minutes
- Cooking time: 5 to 15 minutes

With the texture of steak and the benefits of fish, tuna is a true winner. So is this easy, easy dish. Grill some fresh vegetables at the same time, slice some tomatoes, and call the family to dinner.

2 medium cloves garlic
1 pound tuna steak

Olive oil spray
1 medium lemon, cut into wedges
(optional)

Heat grill on medium-high.

Meanwhile, cut each garlic clove lengthwise into 5 or 6 slices.

Rinse tuna and pat dry with paper towels. Put tuna on a flat surface. With tip of a sharp knife, make one short, ¼-inch-deep cut in fish for each slice of garlic. With your thumb, insert garlic slice into each cut.

Spray both sides of fish with olive oil spray and place on grill. Don't pat or move fish until ready to turn, 3 minutes for medium rare to 10 minutes for well done. Turn fish over and cook for about 2 minutes for medium rare to about 5 minutes for well done.

Serve with lemon wedges.

COOK'S TIP

Vary the flavor of this dish by sprinkling a fresh herb, such as rosemary or dillweed, or some freshly ground pepper over the tuna before grilling it.

(PER SERVING)

Calories 119

Protein 25 g

Carbohydrates 1 g

Cholesterol 53 mg

Total Fat 1 g

Saturated 0 g

Polyunsaturated 0 g

Monounsaturated 0 g

Fiber 0 g

Sodium 42 mg

SEAFOOD

Hawaiian-Style Tuna

Serves 4; 2 cups per serving ■
Preparation time: 10 minutes ■
Cooking time: 19 to 22 minutes ■

With its rainbow of colors, this one-pan dinner looks and tastes great.

1 cup uncooked instant rice

1 tablespoon olive oil

1 medium green bell pepper, diced

1 medium red bell pepper, diced

1 medium yellow pepper, diced

1 large red onion, diced

1 pound tuna or halibut

8-ounce can pineapple chunks in their own juice

6 ounces pineapple juice

1 teaspoon ground ginger (optional)

Cook rice using package directions, omitting salt and margarine.

Meanwhile, heat a large skillet over medium-high heat. Add oil and swirl to coat bottom of skillet. Cook peppers and onion, covered, for 12 minutes, or until they begin to wilt, stirring frequently.

Meanwhile, rinse tuna and pat dry with paper towels. Cut tuna into 1-inch strips.

Add tuna, undrained pineapple, and pineapple juice to skillet and cook, uncovered, for 4 to 7 minutes, or until fish flakes easily when tested with a fork.

Reduce heat to low and add rice and ginger, stirring to mix well. Cook, uncovered, for 2 minutes, or until heated through.

(PER SERVING)

Calories 461

Protein 34 g

Carbohydrates 58 g

Cholesterol 47 mg

Total Fat 10 g

Saturated 2 g

Polyunsaturated 2 g

Monounsaturated 5 g

Fiber 3 g

Sodium 54 mg

Grilled Tuna Niçoise

- Serves 4; 1½ cups per serving
- Preparation time: 15 minutes
- Cooking time: 15 to 20 minutes

Here's a warm version of the popular French dish salade niçoise. *Très bien!*

Olive oil spray

4 4-ounce red potatoes, cut into ⅛-inch slices

9-ounce package frozen no-salt-added French-style green beans (1½ cups)

¼ teaspoon salt

1 pound tuna steaks, ¾ inch thick

1 tablespoon olive oil

1 teaspoon dried basil, crumbled

¼ to ½ teaspoon pepper

8 cherry tomatoes, halved

12 medium or 16 small yellow teardrop tomatoes, halved, or 2 medium yellow tomatoes, diced (about 1 cup)

Whites of 2 large hard-cooked eggs, chopped (optional)

2 teaspoons capers, rinsed and drained

Preheat oven to 400° F. Preheat grill on medium-high.

Lightly spray a baking sheet with olive oil spray. Lay potato slices in a single layer on baking sheet. Lightly spray tops of potatoes with olive oil spray.

Bake for 12 to 15 minutes, or until tender and lightly browned.

Meanwhile, cook green beans using package directions, omitting salt and margarine; drain well. Stir in salt. Cover to keep warm.

Rinse tuna and pat dry with paper towels. Brush one side of tuna with olive oil. Sprinkle with half the basil and half the pepper. Repeat on other side.

Grill tuna for 3 to 5 minutes on each side, or until desired doneness.

To serve, arrange potato slices on each plate. Top with green beans. Stack tuna on top. Serve tomatoes, eggs whites, and capers on the side or sprinkled over tuna.

(PER SERVING)

Calories 376

Protein 34 g

Carbohydrates 38 g

Cholesterol 47 mg

Total Fat 10 g

  Saturated 2 g

  Polyunsaturated 2 g

  Monounsaturated 5 g

Fiber 6 g

Sodium 247 mg

Tuna Casserole with Broccoli and Water Chestnuts

Serves 6; 1½ cups per serving ■
Preparation time: 10 minutes ■
Cooking time: 30 to 32 minutes ■

Everyone needs a tuna casserole recipe. Ours abounds with color, flavor, and crunch.

8 ounces dried or fresh angel hair pasta

Vegetable oil spray

2 6-ounce cans albacore tuna packed in spring or distilled water, rinsed and drained

10.5-ounce can reduced-fat, reduced-sodium cream of chicken soup, undiluted

½ cup sliced canned water chestnuts, rinsed and drained

½ cup no-salt-added canned mushrooms, rinsed and drained (about 4 ounces)

¼ cup fat-free milk

1 to 2 tablespoons plain dry bread crumbs

10-ounce package frozen no-salt-added broccoli florets or green beans or frozen green peas (1½ to 2 cups)

Cook pasta using package directions, omitting salt and oil; drain.

Meanwhile, preheat oven to 375° F.

Spray a 1½-quart casserole dish with vegetable oil spray. Put tuna, soup, water chestnuts, mushrooms, and milk in casserole dish; stir well.

Stir in pasta, sprinkle with bread crumbs, and arrange broccoli around edges of dish.

Bake, uncovered, for 25 minutes, or until warm.

COOK'S TIP ON FRESH PASTA

You can freeze uncooked fresh pasta for up to 1 month. Add it, still frozen, to boiling water; cook for 1 to 2 minutes longer than the package directs. Start timing when you put the pasta in the boiling water. If you let the water return to the boil before you start timing, the pasta may be overcooked.

(PER SERVING)

Calories 266
Protein 20 g
Carbohydrates 40 g
Cholesterol 25 mg
Total Fat 3 g
  Saturated 1 g
  Polyunsaturated 1 g
  Monounsaturated 0 g
Fiber 3 g
Sodium 278 mg

Penne Pasta with Tuna Marinara Sauce

- Serves 5; 1 heaping cup per serving
- Preparation time: 5 minutes
- Cooking time: 15 minutes

Fresh basil and Italian, or flat-leaf, parsley perk up jarred or leftover marinara sauce. Sprinkle some nonfat mozzarella cheese over sautéed zucchini to accompany this simple dish, which tastes even better the second day.

8 ounces dried penne pasta

1 tablespoon extra-virgin olive oil

½ teaspoon bottled minced garlic or 1 medium clove garlic, minced

12-ounce can tuna, packed in spring or distilled water, rinsed and drained

28 ounces low-fat, low-sodium marinara sauce or fresh tomato sauce

1 tablespoon snipped fresh parsley (Italian, or flat-leaf, preferred)

2 leaves fresh basil or 1 teaspoon dried, crumbled

Prepare pasta using package directions, omitting salt and oil; drain well.

Meanwhile, heat a large skillet over medium-high heat. Add oil and swirl to coat bottom of skillet. Cook garlic for 2 minutes.

Add tuna and cook for 1 minute, stirring to break tuna chunks apart.

Stir in remaining ingredients. Cook for 10 minutes, or until sauce is hot.

Stir in pasta and heat for 1 minute.

(PER SERVING)

Calories 357

Protein 24 g

Carbohydrates 45 g

Cholesterol 23 mg

Total Fat 8 g

  Saturated 1 g

  Polyunsaturated —

  Monounsaturated —

Fiber 4 g

Sodium 337 mg

Fish B

Serves 4; 3 ounces f

Preparation time: 5 minutes ■

Cooking time: 15 minutes ■

When the French cook en papillote, *they steam the food in parchment paper. Here we use aluminum foil to provide the same results. Both dinner and cleanup are super quick.*

4 fish fillets, such as sea bass, red snapper, salmon, or trout (about 4 ounces each)

4 medium Italian plum tomatoes or about 2 cups diced seeded tomatoes

Vegetable oil spray

1 teaspoon bottled chopped garlic or 2 medium cloves garlic, chopped

½ teaspoon salt

½ teaspoon crushed red pepper flakes

8 to 12 fresh basil leaves

¼ cup dry white wine (regular or nonalcoholic)

Preheat oven to 375° F or preheat grill on medium. Rinse fish and pat dry with paper towels.

Core tomatoes; slice about ¼ inch thick.

Tear four sheets of aluminum foil, each about 12 x 10 inches. Fold each sheet in half, then open again. Lightly spray with vegetable oil spray. To assemble, place a fillet on right-hand side of each sheet. Spread each fillet with garlic, then sprinkle with salt and crushed red pepper. Add basil and tomatoes. Pour 1 tablespoon wine over each serving. Fold foil over fish. Tightly fold up all three sides of foil to enclose fish.

Bake or grill bundles for about 15 minutes, or until fish flakes easily when tested with a fork.

To serve, carefully unfold one side of foil (being careful not to get a steam burn) and slide contents onto plate.

(PER SERVING)

Calories 133

Protein 22 g

Carbohydrates 3 g

Cholesterol 47 mg

Total Fat 2 g

   Saturated 1 g

    Polyunsaturated 1 g

    Monounsaturated 1 g

Fiber 1 g

Sodium 376 mg

Crumb-Crusted Fish Fillets

- Serves 4; 3 ounces fish per serving
- Preparation time: 15 minutes
- Cooking time: 12 to 15 minutes

This basic fish dish is equally appealing with a crumb topping or Cajun spices. It's so easy to prepare that it's just about foolproof.

Olive oil spray

4 fish fillets, such as orange roughy or halibut, about 1 inch thick (about 4 ounces each)

Topping

¼ cup plain dry bread crumbs

1 tablespoon dried chives or 1 green onion, chopped (green part only)

1 tablespoon light margarine, softened

½ teaspoon salt-free lemon pepper

Sauce

¼ cup fat-free or low-fat plain yogurt

¼ teaspoon salt-free lemon pepper

¼ teaspoon garlic powder

¼ teaspoon onion powder

■ ■ ■

1 small lemon, cut in wedges (optional)

Preheat oven to 425° F. Heavily spray a shallow, 1½-quart baking dish with olive oil spray. Rinse fish and pat dry with paper towels. Put fish in baking dish.

In a small bowl, stir together topping ingredients; sprinkle over fish.

Bake for 12 to 15 minutes, or until fish flakes easily when tested with a fork.

Meanwhile, in a small bowl, stir together sauce ingredients. Spoon over baked fish, and garnish with lemon wedges.

CAJUN BAKED FISH

Omit sauce and lemon. Replace topping with mixture of 1 teaspoon ground cumin, 1 teaspoon chili powder, ½ teaspoon garlic powder, ½ teaspoon onion powder, and

½ teaspoon dried thyme, crumbled. Lightly spray both sides of fish with olive oil spray; sprinkle both sides with the cumin mixture. Spray a 1½-quart baking dish with olive oil spray. Bake as above. (Calories 85; Protein 17 g; Carbohydrates 1 g; Cholesterol 23 mg; Total Fat 1 g; Saturated 0 g; Polyunsaturated 0 g; Monounsaturated 1 g; Fiber 0 g; Sodium 79 mg)

COOK'S TIP ON ORANGE ROUGHY

Orange roughy is usually frozen, then sent to the grocery store and thawed. If you refreeze and rethaw it, the texture will be harmed.

(PER SERVING)

Calories 118
Protein 19 g
Carbohydrates 8 g
Cholesterol 23 mg
Total Fat 1 g
  Saturated 0 g
  Polyunsaturated 0 g
  Monounsaturated 1 g
Fiber 0 g
Sodium 142 mg

Fish with Chunky Creole Sauce

- Serves 4; 3 ounces fish and ¼ cup sauce per serving
- Preparation time: 10 minutes
- Cooking time: 30 to 32 minutes

This mildly seasoned fish with a medley of Creole veggies is wonderful over steamed rice.

Chunky Creole Sauce

1 tablespoon acceptable margarine

1 large tomato, chopped (about 8 ounces)

1 cup frozen chopped green bell pepper or 1 large green bell pepper, chopped

¾ cup thinly sliced celery (1½ medium ribs)

½ cup frozen chopped onion or 1 medium onion, chopped

1 teaspoon bottled minced garlic or 2 medium cloves garlic, minced

½ teaspoon dried thyme, crumbled, or 2 tablespoons finely snipped fresh parsley

½ teaspoon very low sodium or low-sodium Worcestershire sauce

¼ teaspoon sugar

■ ■ ■

4 white fish fillets, such as tilapia, flounder, or snapper (about 4 ounces each)

⅛ teaspoon salt (optional)

(PER SERVING)

Calories 163
Protein 23 g
Carbohydrates 8 g
Cholesterol 60 mg
Total Fat 5 g
  Saturated 1 g
  Polyunsaturated 1 g
  Monounsaturated 2 g
Fiber 2 g
Sodium 155 mg

For sauce, heat a large nonstick skillet over medium-high heat. Melt margarine and swirl to coat bottom of skillet. When margarine is bubbly, add remaining sauce ingredients; bring to a boil. Reduce heat and simmer, covered, for 22 minutes, or until celery is tender.

Meanwhile, rinse fish and pat dry with paper towels. When celery is tender, move vegetable mixture to side of skillet. Add fish; spoon sauce and vegetables over fish. Cook, uncovered, for 6 to 8 minutes, or until fish flakes easily when tested with a fork. Sprinkle with salt.

COOK'S TIP

The sugar reduces the acidity and sharpness of the tomato and gives a mellow taste to the dish.

Scallops Provençal

Serves 4; 1 cup per serving ■
Preparation time: 10 minutes ■
Cooking time: 12 to 15 minutes ■

This recipe is a great example of how to prepare a classic French dinner in minutes and in only one pan.

1 tablespoon extra-virgin olive oil

1 medium to large zucchini, diced (5 to 7 ounces)

1 teaspoon bottled minced garlic or 2 medium cloves garlic, finely chopped

¼ teaspoon dried thyme, crumbled

Pepper to taste

1 pound bay or sea scallops (about 2 cups)

10 to 12 cherry tomatoes

⅓ cup dry white wine (regular or nonalcoholic)

Heat a 12-inch skillet or a Dutch oven over medium-high heat. Add oil and swirl to coat bottom of skillet. Cook zucchini, garlic, thyme, and pepper for 5 to 8 minutes, or until vegetables are crisp-tender, stirring occasionally.

Meanwhile, rinse scallops and pat dry with paper towels. Cut tomatoes in half. Stir scallops, tomatoes, and wine into vegetable mixture. Cook for about 4 minutes for bay scallops or 5 minutes for sea scallops, or until scallops have turned white and zucchini is tender, stirring occasionally.

COOK'S TIP ON SCALLOPS

Bay scallops are much smaller than the sweeter sea scallops and usually cost far less. Watch the scallops carefully—if overcooked, they're rubbery and tough. Once cooked, scallops turn solid white.

(PER SERVING)

Calories 141

Protein 16 g

Carbohydrates 5 g

Cholesterol 37 mg

Total Fat 4 g

Saturated 0 g

Polyunsaturated 0 g

Monounsaturated 3 g

Fiber 1 g

Sodium 182 mg

Pan-Blackened Scallops over Lemon Rice

- Serves 4; 1½ cups per serving
- Preparation time: 10 minutes
- Cooking time: 10 to 12 minutes

If you love spicy food, this dish is for you. The combination of blackening spice and chutney will tantalize your taste buds.

1 cup uncooked instant rice

Juice of 1 medium lemon (about 3 tablespoons)

1 pound sea scallops (about 2 cups)

1 tablespoon olive oil

1 tablespoon blackening spice, divided use

1 teaspoon white pepper, divided use

¼ cup frozen peas

2 tablespoons fresh or bottled chutney

Cook rice using package directions, omitting salt and margarine but adding lemon juice to water.

Rinse scallops and pat dry with paper towels. Put scallops in a medium bowl. Add oil and stir well to coat. Sprinkle half the blackening spice and half the pepper over scallops; stir.

Heat a large nonstick skillet over high heat. Cook scallops for 4 to 5 minutes, or until slightly firm, without stirring. Sprinkle with remaining blackening spice and pepper. Turn over and cook for 5 minutes, or until opaque, without stirring.

Meanwhile, prepare peas using package directions, omitting salt and margarine.

To serve, arrange rice on a serving plate and sprinkle with peas. Place scallops over all. Top with chutney.

(PER SERVING)

Calories 260

Protein 21 g

Carbohydrates 32 g

Cholesterol 37 mg

Total Fat 4 g

  Saturated 1 g

  Polyunsaturated 1 g

  Monounsaturated 3 g

Fiber 1 g

Sodium 437 mg

Barbecue Shrimp Kebabs

Serves 4; 3 ounces shrimp, 1 vegetable skewer, and ½ cup rice per serving ■
Preparation time: 15 minutes ■
Cooking time: 25 minutes ■

Coffee and maple syrup, plus a touch of fire from crushed red pepper flakes, turn ordinary barbecue sauce into something special.

⅔ cup uncooked rice

1 medium red bell pepper, cut lengthwise into fourths

1 medium green bell pepper, cut lengthwise into fourths

2 medium onions, quartered

8 large fresh mushrooms

12 ounces peeled and deveined jumbo shrimp (about 1 pound in the shell)

½ cup barbecue sauce

1 tablespoon brewed coffee

1 tablespoon maple syrup

⅛ to ¼ teaspoon crushed red pepper flakes (optional)

Prepare rice using package directions, omitting salt and margarine.

Meanwhile, preheat grill on medium-high.

Using four metal skewers, alternate peppers, onions, and mushrooms on each. Put shrimp on two more metal skewers. Place all in a single layer in a shallow dish.

In a small bowl, whisk together remaining ingredients. Pour over shrimp and vegetables; turn skewers to coat evenly.

Grill vegetable skewers for 10 minutes, turning every 5 minutes. Add shrimp to grill; cook for 3 minutes, turn, and cook for 2 minutes, or until shrimp turn pink.

Serve shrimp on rice with skewered vegetables on the side.

(PER SERVING)

Calories 309

Protein 22 g

Carbohydrates 48 g

Cholesterol 135 mg

Total Fat 2 g

   Saturated 0 g

   Polyunsaturated 1 g

   Monounsaturated 0 g

Fiber 3 g

Sodium 349 mg

Shrimp Marsala

- Serves 4; 1 cup per serving
- Preparation time: 10 minutes
- Cooking time: 10 to 11 minutes

Shrimp Marsala has it all—savory aroma, the rich flavor of wine and mushrooms, and company-pretty looks. A baked potato and steamed asparagus would go well with this.

1 pound uncooked peeled and deveined colossal shrimp (about 1⅓ pounds shrimp in the shell)

2 tablespoons all-purpose flour

1 tablespoon extra-virgin olive oil

5 ounces presliced fresh mushrooms

½ cup marsala

Fresh parsley, snipped (optional)

Rinse shrimp; pat dry with paper towels. Sprinkle flour over shrimp, shaking off excess.

Heat a large skillet over medium-high heat. Add oil and swirl to coat bottom of skillet. When oil is hot, cook shrimp for 2 minutes. Turn shrimp over.

Add mushrooms and marsala to skillet. Increase heat to high and cook for 5 to 7 minutes, stirring occasionally, until sauce has thickened to a consistency almost like melted caramels.

To serve, place equal amounts of each on four plates and top with parsley.

(PER SERVING)

Calories 168

Protein 19 g

Carbohydrates 6 g

Cholesterol 135 mg

Total Fat 5 g

  Saturated 1 g

  Polyunsaturated 1 g

  Monounsaturated 3 g

Fiber 1 g

Sodium 134 mg

SEAFOOD

Spanish Shrimp

Serves 4; 1¼ cups per serving ■
Preparation time: 10 minutes ■
Cooking time: 23 to 24 minutes ■

The aroma of this dish will attract your family to the table. Serve this colorful entrée with rice—perhaps topped with a dollop of nonfat sour cream—so you can enjoy every bit of the sauce. For a Tex-Mex version, cut the vegetables into smaller pieces and wrap the finished mixture in flour tortillas. Again, a little sour cream is a good addition.

1 tablespoon plus 1 teaspoon olive oil

2 medium yellow or white onions, each cut into eighths (Spanish preferred)

3 cups frozen red, yellow, and green bell pepper strips or 1 medium red bell pepper, 1 medium yellow bell pepper, and 1 medium green bell pepper, cut into 1-inch strips

1 teaspoon bottled chopped garlic or 2 medium cloves garlic, chopped

½ pound uncooked peeled and deveined medium shrimp (about 20) (about 11 ounces shrimp in shell)

¼ cup lime juice (2 to 3 medium limes)

1 tablespoon snipped fresh cilantro

¼ teaspoon crushed red pepper flakes, or to taste

Heat a large skillet over medium heat. Add oil and swirl to coat bottom of skillet. Sauté onions, peppers, and garlic, uncovered, for 15 minutes, stirring occasionally.

Stir in remaining ingredients. Cook for 7 to 8 minutes, or until shrimp turns pink, stirring frequently.

COOK'S TIP ON BUYING SHRIMP

Shrimp loses about 25 percent of its weight when peeled and deveined. Then the peeled shrimp loses another one fourth of its original weight when cooked. If you start with 12 ounces of raw shrimp in the shell, you'll wind up with about 6 ounces of cooked, peeled shrimp.

(PER SERVING)

Calories 144

Protein 13 g

Carbohydrates 11 g

Cholesterol 86 mg

Total Fat 6 g

   Saturated 1 g

   Polyunsaturated 1 g

   Monounsaturated 4 g

Fiber 2 g

Sodium 89 mg

Mixed Kebabs

- Serves 4; 3 ounces per serving
- Preparation time: 10 minutes
- Marinating time: 6 to 8 minutes
- Cooking time: 6 to 8 minutes

Whether your family craves Italian, Tex-Mex, or Asian food tonight, this simple standby with its triple combination of meat and seafood and its choice of marinades will come to your rescue. To save time, buy preskewered kebabs at the supermarket. Be sure to choose the leanest ones.

Kebabs

12 large shrimp in shells, peeled and deveined (about 6 ounces)

⅓ pound boneless, skinless chicken breast halves, all visible fat removed

⅓ pound sirloin steak, all visible fat removed

Italian Marinade

2 teaspoons balsamic vinegar

1 teaspoon dried oregano, crumbled

1 teaspoon bottled minced garlic or 2 medium cloves garlic, minced

1 teaspoon olive oil

Tex-Mex Marinade

2 teaspoons lime juice

1 teaspoon bottled minced garlic or 2 medium cloves garlic, minced

1 teaspoon acceptable vegetable oil

½ teaspoon garlic powder

Asian Marinade

2 teaspoons light soy sauce

1 teaspoon bottled minced garlic or 2 medium cloves garlic, minced

1 teaspoon acceptable vegetable oil

½ teaspoon toasted sesame oil

Rinse shrimp and chicken and pat dry with paper towels. Cut chicken into ¾-inch cubes. Cut beef into 1-inch cubes.

In a large airtight plastic bag, combine ingredients for your choice of one marinade. Add shrimp, chicken, and beef; seal and turn to coat.

Marinate for 5 to 10 minutes at room temperature.

Meanwhile, preheat grill.

Remove shrimp, chicken, and beef from marinade;

discard marinade. Thread kebab ingredients alternately on four 10-inch metal skewers, or thread chicken on one skewer, beef on one skewer, and shrimp on two skewers.

Grill kebabs over medium-high heat for 3 to 4 minutes per side, or until shrimp turns pink and is cooked through, chicken is no longer pink in center, and beef is done to your liking.

Cook's Tip

If you want your steak cubes well done, use ¾-inch cubes. The 1-inch size will give you medium-well in this recipe.

Cook's Tip

The nutrient analysis is for Italian or Tex-Mex marinade. If you select the Asian marinade, the sodium increases to 131 mg. All the other nutrients remain the same.

(PER SERVING)
Calories 112
Protein 20 g
Carbohydrates 0 g
Cholesterol 75 mg
Total Fat 3 g
  Saturated 1 g
  Polyunsaturated 0 g
  Monounsaturated 1 g
Fiber 0 g
Sodium 66 mg

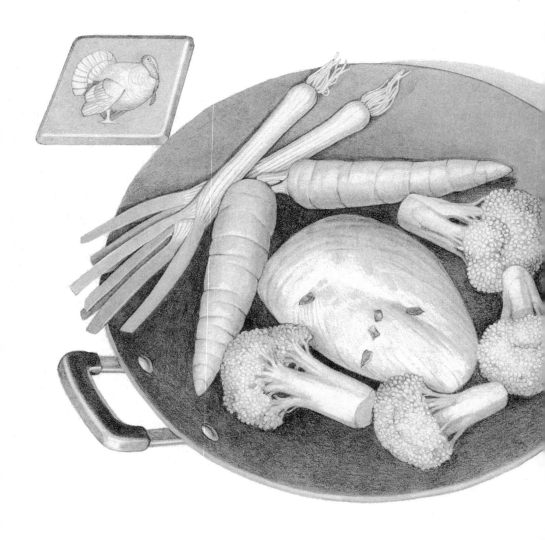

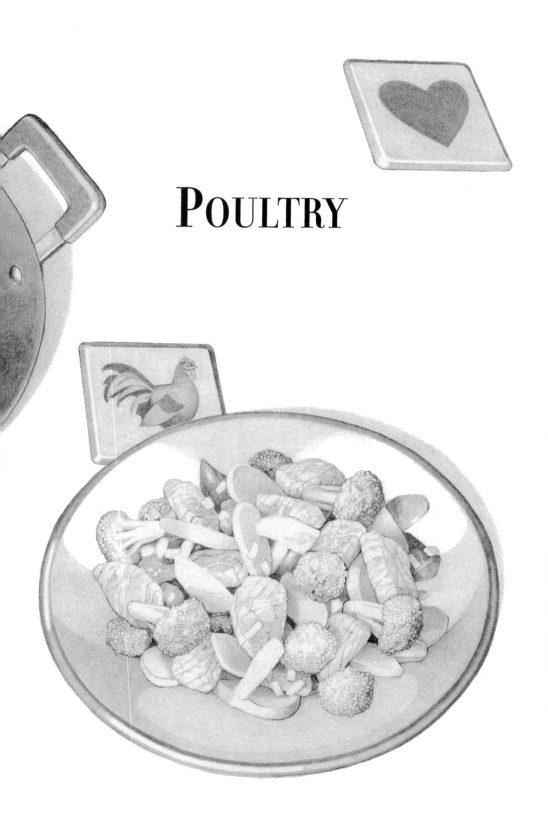

POULTRY

■ ■ ■

Slow-Cooker Chicken
and Bell Pepper Stew

Crispy Chicken with Creamy Gravy

Roasted Chicken Breasts
with Garlic Gravy

Sun-Dried Tomato Pesto Chicken
and Pasta

   Basil-Parmesan Pesto Chicken
   and Pasta

Orange-Barbecue Chicken Chunks

Spicy Honey-Kissed Chicken

Chicken, Spinach, and Pasta
Casserole

Grilled Chicken with Green Chiles
and Cheese

   Italian Grilled Chicken

   Barbecued Chicken Dijon

Two-Way Border Chicken

Curried Chicken and Cauliflower

Butter Bean, Chicken,
and Vegetable Stew

Chicken and Shrimp Stir-Fry

Chicken and Vegetable Stir-Fry

   Italian Stir-Fry

Bloody Mary Chicken and Rice

Dilled Chicken with Mushrooms
and Rice

Bell Pepper Chicken and Noodles

Chicken Fajita Pasta
with Chipotle Alfredo Sauce

Greek Chicken Thighs

Polynesian Chicken
in a Slow Cooker

   Mediterranean Chicken
   in a Slow Cooker

Southwestern-Style Roasted
Chicken

Sour Cream Chicken Enchiladas

Curried Chicken, Pasta,
and Vegetable Casserole

   Curried Pasta and Vegetable
   Casserole

   Chicken, Pasta, and Vegetable
   Casserole

   Pasta and Vegetable Casserole

Lemongrass Chicken with Snow
Peas and Jasmine Rice

Creamed Chicken and Vegetables

   Creamed Tuna and Vegetables

Turkey and Broccoli Stir-Fry

   Vegetarian Stir-Fry

Turkey Cutlets with Two Sauces

Italian Bean Stew with Turkey
and Ham

Grilled Turkey Cutlets
with Pineapple

Turkey Breast with Cranberry Sage
Stuffing

■ ■ ■

Slow-Cooker Chicken and Bell Pepper Stew

Serves 4; 1¼ cups per serving ■
Preparation time: 10 minutes ■
Cooking time: 4 hours ■

❶

The beans break apart and almost disappear, giving this stew a rich, thick consistency.

1½ pounds skinless chicken breasts with ribs, all visible fat removed

2 cups frozen chopped green bell pepper or 2 large green bell peppers, coarsely chopped (about 1 pound)

1½ cups frozen chopped onion or 3 medium onions, coarsely chopped (yellow preferred)

1½ cups hot tap water

15-ounce can no-salt-added cannellini beans, rinsed and drained

14.5-ounce can no-salt-added diced tomatoes

1½ teaspoons ground cumin

1½ teaspoons sugar

1 teaspoon dried oregano, crumbled

½ teaspoon salt

½ teaspoon ground cumin

½ cup finely snipped fresh cilantro (optional)

Rinse chicken and pat dry with paper towels. Put in slow cooker.

In a large bowl, stir together bell peppers, onion, water, beans, undrained tomatoes, 1½ teaspoons cumin, sugar, and oregano. Pour over chicken.

Cook on high for 4 hours, or until chicken begins to fall off bone. Remove chicken with slotted spoon. Using two forks, shred chicken, discarding ribs. Return chicken to slow cooker.

Stir in salt and ½ teaspoon cumin.

To serve, ladle into bowls and sprinkle each serving with cilantro.

COOK'S TIP

For this recipe, be sure to use chicken breasts with the bone in. They provide not only a lot of flavor but the right texture; boneless breasts become overcooked.

(PER SERVING)

Calories 275

Protein 32 g

Carbohydrates 29 g

Cholesterol 66 mg

Total Fat 4 g

  Saturated 1 g

  Polyunsaturated 1 g

  Monounsaturated 1 g

Fiber 7 g

Sodium 373 mg

Crispy Chicken with Creamy Gravy

- Serves 4; 3 ounces chicken and ¼ cup gravy per serving
- Preparation time: 10 minutes
- Cooking time: 10 to 13 minutes

Recapture Sunday lunches from the past by making this crispy-coated chicken and extra gravy to top low-fat mashed potatoes.

4 boneless, skinless chicken breast halves (about 4 ounces each), all visible fat removed

2 tablespoons all-purpose flour

Egg substitute equivalent to 1 egg, or 1 large egg

¼ cup unsalted cracker crumbs (about 7 crackers)

1 teaspoon salt-free all-purpose seasoning

Vegetable oil spray

1 tablespoon acceptable vegetable oil

½ cup bottled fat-free chicken gravy

½ cup fat-free milk

1 tablespoon all-purpose flour

Rinse chicken and pat dry with paper towels. Put chicken smooth side up between two sheets of plastic wrap. Using a tortilla press or smooth side of a meat mallet, lightly flatten chicken, being careful not to tear meat.

Put 2 tablespoons flour in a large airtight plastic bag. Add chicken and shake to coat.

Pour egg substitute into bag and shake to coat.

Combine cracker crumbs and all-purpose seasoning in a shallow bowl. Roll chicken in mixture. Lightly spray both sides with vegetable oil spray.

Heat a large nonstick skillet over medium heat. Add oil and swirl to coat bottom of skillet. Cook chicken meaty side down for 4 to 5 minutes, or until browned on bottom.

Turn chicken over and cook for 4 to 5 minutes, or until no longer pink in center. Transfer chicken to a platter and cover with aluminum foil to keep warm.

Put chicken gravy, milk, and 1 tablespoon flour in skillet; whisk thoroughly. Cook over medium heat until thick and bubbly, 2 to 3 minutes, stirring occasionally. Spoon over chicken.

(PER SERVING)

Calories 240

Protein 29 g

Carbohydrates 13 g

Cholesterol 67 mg

Total Fat 7 g

  Saturated 1 g

  Polyunsaturated 3 g

  Monounsaturated 2 g

Fiber 0 g

Sodium 288 mg

Roasted Chicken Breasts
with Garlic Gravy

Serves 4; 3 ounces chicken and scant ½ cup gravy per serving ■
Preparation time: 15 minutes ■
Microwave time: 1 minute ■
Cooking time: 22 minutes ■

This yummy chicken and gravy combination goes well with just about any side dish.

Vegetable oil spray

2 large, plump whole garlic bulbs

1 tablespoon olive oil

4 boneless, skinless chicken breast halves, all visible fat removed (about 4 ounces each)

1 teaspoon dried thyme, crumbled

¼ teaspoon freshly ground pepper

½ teaspoon salt (divided use)

2 cups low-sodium chicken broth

1 tablespoon all-purpose flour

Preheat oven to 400° F. Spray a jelly-roll pan with vegetable oil spray.

Cut about ¼ inch off top of garlic bulbs to create a flat top and expose middle cloves. Microwave on a micro-wave-safe plate at 100 percent power (high) for 1 minute.

Separate cloves of garlic and peel off skins (they should slip off very easily). Heap garlic on jelly-roll pan, drizzle garlic with olive oil, then spread garlic toward edges of pan.

Rinse chicken and pat dry with paper towels. Sprinkle both sides of chicken with thyme, pepper, and ¼ tea-spoon salt. Put chicken in middle of pan.

Bake for 20 minutes, or until no longer pink in center. If small garlic cloves go beyond golden stage, remove them. Transfer chicken to serving platter or plates; put garlic in a large skillet. Crush garlic with back of a spoon or fork. Add remaining ¼ teaspoon salt.

In a jar with a tight-fitting lid, combine broth and flour. Cover and shake until completely blended. Add to garlic and bring to a boil over medium heat, stirring con-stantly and continuing to break up garlic. When sauce thickens and boils, about 2 minutes, pour over chicken.

(PER SERVING)

Calories 215

Protein 29 g

Carbohydrates 7 g

Cholesterol 74 mg

Total Fat 7 g

  Saturated 1 g

  Polyunsaturated 1 g

  Monounsaturated 4 g

Fiber 0 g

Sodium 415 mg

Sun-Dried Tomato Pesto Chicken and Pasta

- Serves 4; 3 ounces chicken and 1 cup pasta per serving
- Preparation time: 10 minutes
- Cooking time: 12 minutes

This fantastically easy recipe uses bottled sun-dried tomato pesto to cut your prep time.

4 boneless, skinless chicken breast halves, all visible fat removed (about 4 ounces each)

Vegetable oil spray

¼ cup bottled sun-dried tomato pesto

2 tablespoons water

2 tablespoons dry red wine (regular or nonalcoholic)

1 tablespoon balsamic vinegar

1 tablespoon plus 1½ teaspoons dried basil, crumbled

¼ teaspoon salt

9 ounces refrigerated fat-free angel hair pasta

Put hot tap water for pasta on to boil, covering pan. Rinse chicken and pat dry with paper towels.

Heat a large nonstick skillet over medium-high heat. Remove from heat and spray with vegetable oil spray. Return to heat and cook chicken for 2 minutes on each side.

Meanwhile, in a small mixing bowl, whisk together remaining ingredients except pasta. Pour over chicken. Reduce heat and simmer, covered, for 6 to 8 minutes, or until chicken is no longer pink in center.

When water for pasta comes to a boil, cook pasta using package directions, omitting salt and oil; don't overcook. Drain well.

To serve, place pasta on serving platter, arrange chicken on top, and spoon sauce over all.

BASIL-PARMESAN PESTO CHICKEN AND PASTA

Replace sun-dried tomato pesto with basil-Parmesan pesto, dry red wine with dry white wine, and balsamic vinegar with lemon juice. (Calories 367; Protein 33 g; Carbohydrates 37 g; Cholesterol 67 mg; Total Fat 9 g; Saturated 2 g; Polyunsaturated —; Monounsaturated —; Fiber 3 g; Sodium 293 mg)

COOK'S TIP

If you don't have a tight-fitting lid to use while preparing this dish, tightly cover the skillet with aluminum foil. This will keep the moisture in, helping the sauce get a marinara-like consistency.

COOK'S TIP ON WHITE-MEAT CHICKEN

Remember that white meat can overcook quickly. Cook breasts just until they are barely pink in the middle; then remove them from the heat. Residual heat will finish cooking the breasts.

(PER SERVING)
Calories 319
Protein 32 g
Carbohydrates 39 g
Cholesterol 67 mg
Total Fat 3 g
  Saturated 1 g
  Polyunsaturated 1 g
  Monounsaturated 1 g
Fiber 3 g
Sodium 249 mg

Orange-Barbecue Chicken Chunks

- Serves 4; ½ cup per serving (plus 2 cups reserved)
- Preparation time: 5 minutes
- Cooking time: 7 to 8 minutes

Here's the answer when you have to have a kid-pleasing entrée in next to no time. This recipe even gives you a bonus—planned-overs to use in Asian Chicken and Wild Rice Salad (page 84).

2 pounds boneless, skinless chicken breasts or turkey breast tender-loins, all visible fat removed

Vegetable oil spray

½ cup barbecue sauce

½ cup all-fruit marmalade or spread, such as orange, apricot, or plum

1 teaspoon powdered ginger (optional)

Rinse chicken and pat dry with paper towels. Cut chicken into bite-size pieces.

Heat a large skillet over medium-high heat. Remove from heat and spray with vegetable oil spray. Cook chicken for 3 to 4 minutes, or until tender and no longer pink in center, stirring occasionally.

Stir in remaining ingredients. Cook until heated through, about 3 minutes, stirring constantly.

Cook's Tip on Cooking Oil Spray

Unless you're using cast iron, heat your pot or pan, re-move it from the heat, then lightly spray it with veg-etable oil spray. Spraying after heating the pan prevents the oil from baking into the pan's surface. The baked-in coating of oil tends to cause foods to stick if it is not cleaned off completely after each use—not an easy thing to do.

(PER SERVING)

Calories 183

Protein 25 g

Carbohydrates 14 g

Cholesterol 67 mg

Total Fat 3 g

  Saturated 1 g

  Polyunsaturated 1 g

  Monounsaturated 1 g

Fiber 0 g

Sodium 200 mg

Spicy Honey-Kissed Chicken

Serves 4; 1 cup per serving ■
Preparation time: 5 minutes ■
Cooking time: 5 to 8 minutes ■

Cumin, sage, and ginger spice up the rub that gives this chicken its distinctive flavor.

Rub

1 teaspoon ground cumin

½ teaspoon rubbed or crumbled sage

½ teaspoon ground ginger

¼ to ½ teaspoon freshly ground pepper

½ teaspoon salt

■ ■ ■

1 pound boneless, skinless chicken breasts, all visible fat removed

1 tablespoon acceptable vegetable oil

3 tablespoons lemon juice

1 tablespoon honey

1 tablespoon light soy sauce

In a small dish, combine rub ingredients. Rinse chicken and pat dry with paper towels. Rub mixture all over chicken. Cut into strips about ½ inch wide.

Heat a large skillet (preferably nonstick) over medium-high heat. Add oil and swirl to coat bottom of skillet. Cook chicken until nearly cooked through, 3 to 5 minutes, stirring often.

Meanwhile, in a small bowl, whisk together remaining ingredients. Stir into chicken, increase heat to high, and cook for 1 to 2 minutes, or until chicken has just cooked through.

COOK'S TIP

If you prefer to leave the breasts whole instead of cutting them into strips, reduce the cooking temperature to medium and increase the cooking time to about 15 minutes before adding the lemon juice mixture.

(PER SERVING)

Calories 197
Protein 27 g
Carbohydrates 6 g
Cholesterol 73 mg
Total Fat 7 g
  Saturated 1 g
  Polyunsaturated 3 g
  Monounsaturated 2 g
Fiber 0 g
Sodium 455 mg

Chicken, Spinach, and Pasta Casserole

- Serves 8; 1 cup per serving
- Preparation time: 20 minutes
- Cooking time: 45 minutes

Tantalize your guests with this delightful dish. It combines spinach and three cheeses with tender chicken morsels and, surprisingly, fresh cilantro.

Vegetable oil spray

8 cups hot tap water

4 ounces chèvre (goat cheese)

4 ounces crumbled nonfat feta cheese, rinsed

¼ cup fat-free evaporated milk (½ of a large can)

½ cup fat-free or low-fat plain yogurt

Egg substitute equivalent to 1 egg, or 1 large egg

¼ teaspoon white pepper

1 pound boneless, skinless chicken breasts, all visible fat removed

8 ounces dried angel hair pasta

10 ounces frozen spinach, thawed and squeezed dry

¼ teaspoon ground nutmeg

2 tablespoons snipped fresh cilantro

⅔ cup grated nonfat mozzarella-style soy cheese or nonfat or part-skim mozzarella cheese (3 ounces)

Preheat oven to 350° F. Spray a 2-quart casserole dish with vegetable oil spray.

In a stockpot, bring water to a boil, covered, over high heat.

Meanwhile, cut chèvre into eight pieces and put in a large bowl; set aside.

In a small bowl, whisk together feta, milk, yogurt, egg substitute, and pepper.

Rinse chicken and pat dry with paper towels. Cut into strips about 1 inch wide and 4 inches long.

Cook pasta in boiling water for 1 minute. Before draining pasta, remove ½ cup cooking water and stir into chèvre. Drain pasta, add to chèvre, and stir well.

To assemble, spread half the pasta mixture in casserole dish. Scatter spinach over top, sprinkle with nutmeg, and pour half the feta mixture over all. Cover with remaining pasta. Arrange chicken and cilantro on top.

Pour remaining feta mixture over chicken, making sure to cover all surfaces. Sprinkle with soy cheese.

Bake, covered, for 35 minutes. Uncover and bake for 10 minutes, or until bubbly.

TIME-SAVER

Substituting 12 ounces of boneless, skinless cooked chicken strips for the raw chicken not only saves on preparation time but also reduces the cooking time by about 25 minutes. Assemble the casserole as directed. Bake, covered, for 10 minutes; uncover and bake for 10 minutes, or until bubbly.

(PER SERVING)

Calories 282

Protein 28 g

Carbohydrates 28 g

Cholesterol 41 mg

Total Fat 6 g

  Saturated 3 g

  Polyunsaturated 1 g

  Monounsaturated 2 g

Fiber 2 g

Sodium 472 mg

Grilled Chicken with Green Chiles and Cheese

- Serves 4; 3 ounces chicken per serving
- Preparation time: 10 minutes
- Cooking time: 8 to 10 minutes

With this southwestern-style dish and the two variations below, you can break out of a plain-chicken rut!

4 boneless, skinless chicken breast halves (about 4 ounces each), all visible fat removed

Olive oil spray

1 teaspoon chili powder

¼ cup diced canned green chiles, rinsed and drained

¼ cup shredded reduced-fat Cheddar cheese (about 1 ounce)

Preheat grill on medium-high.

Rinse chicken and pat dry with paper towels. Spray one side of chicken with olive oil spray and sprinkle with half the chili powder. Turn breasts over and repeat.

Grill chicken for 4 to 5 minutes; turn over. Spread 1 tablespoon green chiles and 1 tablespoon cheese on each breast. Grill for 4 to 5 minutes, or until chicken is no longer pink in center.

ITALIAN GRILLED CHICKEN

Replace chili powder with dried oregano, crumbled; green chiles with 1 thinly sliced medium bell pepper, any color, and 1 thinly sliced medium onion; and ¼ cup Cheddar cheese with 2 tablespoons shredded or grated Parmesan cheese. Sprinkle oregano over chicken. While chicken grills, heat a medium skillet over medium-high heat. Add 1 teaspoon olive oil and swirl to coat bottom of skillet. Sauté bell pepper and onion for 2 to 3 minutes, or until tender. To serve, place chicken on a platter and top with peppers and onions. Sprinkle with Parmesan. (Calories 168; Protein 26 g; Carbohydrates 4 g; Cholesterol 69 mg; Total Fat 5 g; Saturated 1 g; Polyunsaturated 1 g; Monounsaturated 2 g; Fiber 1 g; Sodium 108 mg)

BARBECUED CHICKEN DIJON

Replace chili powder with dried rosemary, crushed; replace green chiles and cheese with ¼ cup low-sodium barbecue sauce and 1 teaspoon flavored Dijon mustard, such as horseradish, orange, or honey. Sprinkle chicken with rosemary. While chicken cooks, stir together barbecue sauce and mustard. When chicken is no longer pink in center, brush each side with sauce mixture; grill for 30 seconds on each side to warm sauce. (Calories 147; Protein 24 g; Carbohydrates 5 g; Cholesterol 67 mg; Total Fat 3 g; Saturated 1 g; Polyunsaturated 1 g; Monounsaturated 1 g; Fiber 0 g; Sodium 178 mg)

(PER SERVING)

Calories 156

Protein 27 g

Carbohydrates 1 g

Cholesterol 71 mg

Total Fat 4 g

   Saturated 2 g

   Polyunsaturated 1 g

   Monounsaturated 1 g

Fiber 0 g

Sodium 110 mg

Two-Way Border Chicken

- Serves 4; 3 ounces chicken, ½ cup rice, and ⅔ cup sauce per serving (plus 4 chicken breast halves and 1½ cups sauce reserved)
- Preparation time: 15 minutes
- Cooking time: 20 minutes

 ❶

After enjoying this chicken dish with turmeric-colored rice, you can look forward to an even easier dinner of Yucatecan Wraps (page 100) made from the planned-overs.

2 14.5-ounce cans no-salt-added diced tomatoes, undrained

2 tablespoons lime juice (1 to 2 medium limes)

1- to 1½-ounce package taco seasoning mix

2 teaspoons sugar

1 teaspoon dried oregano, crumbled

1 teaspoon red hot-pepper sauce

8 boneless, skinless chicken breast halves, all visible fat removed (about 4 ounces each)

⅜ cup uncooked rice

¼ teaspoon turmeric

2 tablespoons extra-virgin olive oil

1 teaspoon sugar

2 tablespoons snipped fresh cilantro

In a large bowl, combine undrained tomatoes, lime juice, taco seasoning, 2 teaspoons sugar, oregano, and red hot-pepper sauce.

Rinse chicken and pat dry with paper towels; put chicken in a Dutch oven. Pour tomato mixture over chicken. Bring to a boil over high heat; stir. Reduce heat and simmer, covered, for 20 minutes, stirring occasionally.

Meanwhile, cook rice using package directions, omitting salt and margarine and adding turmeric.

When chicken is done, stir in olive oil and 1 teaspoon sugar. Remove four breasts and 1½ cups sauce. Refrigerate and reserve for Yucatecan Wraps.

To serve, spoon rice onto serving platter, arrange chicken breasts around edge, and pour remaining 2½ cups sauce evenly over chicken pieces. Sprinkle cilantro over chicken.

(PER SERVING)

Calories 351

Protein 31 g

Carbohydrates 37 g

Cholesterol 73 mg

Total Fat 8 g

  Saturated 2 g

  Polyunsaturated 1 g

  Monounsaturated 4 g

Fiber 2 g

Sodium 432 mg

Curried Chicken and Cauliflower

Serves 4; 1 cup per serving ■
Preparation time: 15 minutes ■
Cooking time: 16 to 19 minutes ■

Turn ordinary chicken and cauliflower into a flavor sensation with curry powder and tangy yogurt. Serve over couscous, noodles, or rice.

1 pound boneless, skinless chicken breasts, all visible fat removed

1 teaspoon acceptable vegetable oil

¼ cup frozen chopped onion or ½ medium onion, thinly sliced

1 teaspoon bottled minced garlic or 2 medium cloves garlic, minced

2 cups bite-size pieces of cauliflower (1 medium head)

1 cup low-sodium chicken broth

1 teaspoon curry powder

¼ teaspoon turmeric (optional)

¼ teaspoon salt

⅛ teaspoon pepper

¼ cup water

3 tablespoons all-purpose flour

½ cup fat-free or low-fat plain yogurt

Rinse chicken and pat dry with paper towels. Cut chicken into ¾-inch cubes.

Heat a large nonstick skillet over medium-high heat. Add oil and swirl to coat bottom of skillet. Cook onion and garlic for 2 to 3 minutes, or until onion is translucent, stirring occasionally. Push to one side of skillet.

Add chicken and cook for 4 to 5 minutes, or until chicken is no longer pink in center, stirring occasionally.

Stir in cauliflower, broth, curry powder, turmeric, salt, and pepper; bring to a boil over high heat. Reduce heat to medium-low and cook, covered, for 5 to 6 minutes, or until cauliflower is tender. Increase heat to medium-high.

In a small bowl, whisk together water and flour. Add to skillet and cook, uncovered, for 2 to 3 minutes, or until mixture is thickened, stirring occasionally. Reduce heat to low.

In a small bowl, whisk together a small amount of warm chicken mixture and yogurt. Stir into pan and cook, uncovered, for 1 to 2 minutes, or until warmed through, stirring occasionally.

(PER SERVING)

Calories 204

Protein 28 g

Carbohydrates 11 g

Cholesterol 67 mg

Total Fat 5 g

    Saturated 1 g

    Polyunsaturated 1 g

    Monounsaturated 1 g

Fiber 2 g

Sodium 267 mg

Butter Bean, Chicken, and Vegetable Stew

- Serves 6; 1⅓ cups per serving
- Preparation time: 20 minutes
- Slow-cooker time: 3 to 4 hours on high or 8 to 9 hours on low *or*
  Cooking time: 1 hour

You can prepare this Southern meal either in a slow cooker while you work or run errands, or on top of the stove. Serve with low-fat, low-sodium corn bread.

1½ pounds boneless, skinless chicken breasts, all visible fat removed

4 cups low-sodium chicken broth

16-ounce bag frozen butter beans (lima beans)

2 small turnips, peeled and cubed (8 ounces)

2 ribs celery, cut into ½-inch slices (about 1 cup)

2 medium carrots, cut into ½-inch slices (about 1½ cups)

2 teaspoons onion powder

1 teaspoon garlic powder

1 teaspoon dried thyme, crumbled

¼ to ½ teaspoon salt

½ teaspoon liquid smoke

¼ teaspoon crushed red pepper flakes (optional)

⅛ to ¼ teaspoon black pepper

Rinse chicken and pat dry with paper towels. Cut chicken into 1-inch cubes.

Combine all ingredients in a 3½- to 4-quart slow cooker. Cook, covered, on high for 3 to 4 hours or on low for 8 to 9 hours. To prepare on stovetop, combine all ingredients in a Dutch oven. Bring to a boil over high heat. Reduce heat to medium-low and cook, covered, for 30 to 45 minutes, or until beans are tender.

COOK'S TIP ON BUTTER BEANS

Depending on who you ask, "butter beans" is the Southern name for dried lima beans, the name of a variety of lima bean grown primarily in the South, or another name for Fordhook lima beans. Whatever you call them, you'll enjoy them in this dish.

(PER SERVING)

Calories 275

Protein 32 g

Carbohydrates 26 g

Cholesterol 67 mg

Total Fat 3 g

  Saturated 1 g

  Polyunsaturated 1 g

  Monounsaturated 1 g

Fiber 5 g

Sodium 398 mg

Chicken and Shrimp Stir-Fry

Serves 4; 1 cup per serving ■
Preparation time: 10 minutes ■
Cooking time: 5 to 8 minutes ■

Either chicken and snow peas or shrimp and snow peas is a classic combination. Here you get all three. Serve this dish with rice and tossed salad with Far East Dressing (page 93).

8 ounces boneless, skinless chicken breasts, all visible fat removed

Vegetable oil spray

2 teaspoons acceptable vegetable oil

2 teaspoons bottled chopped garlic or 4 medium cloves garlic, chopped

½ teaspoon crushed red pepper flakes

9 ounces uncooked peeled large shrimp (thawed if frozen) (about 12 ounces in the shell)

8 ounces fresh or frozen no-salt-added snow peas

½ teaspoon salt

Rinse chicken and pat dry with paper towels. Cut chicken crosswise into ¼-inch strips.

Heat a large nonstick skillet over medium-high heat. Remove from heat and spray with vegetable oil spray. Add oil and swirl to coat bottom of skillet. Cook garlic and crushed red pepper for about 30 seconds, or until garlic is aromatic.

Add chicken and shrimp; increase heat to high. Cook for about 2 minutes, stirring constantly.

If using fresh snow peas, cook chicken and shrimp for 2 more minutes before adding peas. Cook, uncovered, for 2 minutes with peas.

If using frozen snow peas, add to chicken and shrimp and cook, covered, for 2 minutes. Uncover and cook for 2 minutes.

Stir in salt.

(PER SERVING)

Calories 163

Protein 24 g

Carbohydrates 5 g

Cholesterol 101 mg

Total Fat 5 g

  Saturated 1 g

  Polyunsaturated 2 g

  Monounsaturated 1 g

Fiber 1 g

Sodium 390 mg

Chicken and Vegetable Stir-Fry

- Serves 4; 1 heaping cup per serving
- Preparation time: 10 minutes
- Cooking time: 7 to 10 minutes

This basic stir-fry recipe gives you many options. You can choose between the Asian and Italian flavorings and vary the meat. (See Italian Stir-Fry and Cook's Tip, below.) Save even more time by using precut vegetables or no-salt-added frozen mixed vegetables (no need to thaw). Even if you make only half of this recipe, you'll probably want the entire amount of sauce.

Sauce

2 tablespoons water

1 tablespoon bottled low-sodium stir-fry sauce

1 teaspoon cornstarch

■ ■ ■

1 pound boneless, skinless chicken breasts, all visible fat removed

1 teaspoon acceptable vegetable oil

1 cup broccoli florets, cut into 1-inch pieces

½ cup sliced red bell pepper

½ cup thinly sliced carrots

½ cup no-salt-added canned baby corn, rinsed, drained, and cut into bite-size pieces

2 green onions, sliced (about ¼ cup)

1 teaspoon bottled minced garlic or 2 medium cloves garlic, minced

For sauce, in a small bowl, stir together all ingredients; set aside.

Rinse chicken and pat dry with paper towels. Thinly slice chicken.

Heat a wok or large skillet over medium-high heat. Add oil and swirl to coat bottom. Cook chicken for 3 to 4 minutes, or until no longer pink in center, stirring occasionally.

Add remaining ingredients and cook for 3 to 4 minutes, or until vegetables are tender-crisp, stirring frequently.

Push chicken mixture aside, making a well in center of wok. Add sauce mixture; stir chicken mixture into sauce. Cook for 1 to 2 minutes, or until sauce has thickened, stirring occasionally.

Italian Stir-Fry

Prepare as directed above except replace sauce mixture with 3 tablespoons low-sodium chicken broth, 1 teaspoon cornstarch, and ½ teaspoon dried oregano, crumbled; replace vegetable oil with olive oil; and replace carrots and corn with ½ cup sliced fresh asparagus and ½ cup sliced zucchini. Add 1 medium sliced Italian plum tomato when adding sauce mixture. Serves 4; 1¼ cups per serving. (Calories 167; Protein 26 g; Carbohydrates 6 g; Cholesterol 67 mg; Total Fat 4 g; Saturated 1 g; Polyunsaturated 1 g; Monounsaturated 2 g; Fiber 2 g; Sodium 73 mg)

Cook's Tip

Substitute 1 pound of any of the following for chicken (remember to remove all visible fat before slicing): boneless round steak, thinly sliced; pork loin chops or pork tenderloin, thinly sliced; shark, halibut, or other firm-fleshed fish, cut into ¾-inch cubes; bay scallops; or 10 ounces reduced-fat firm tofu, cut into ¾-inch cubes.

(PER SERVING)

Calories 171

Protein 26 g

Carbohydrates 6 g

Cholesterol 67 mg

Total Fat 4 g

  Saturated 1 g

  Polyunsaturated 1 g

  Monounsaturated 1 g

Fiber 2 g

Sodium 153 mg

Bloody Mary Chicken and Rice

- Serves 5; 1 cup chicken mixture and 1 scant cup rice per serving
- Preparation time: 10 minutes
- Cooking time: 19 minutes
- Standing time: 2 to 5 minutes

Spicy Bloody Mary mix supplies most of the seasoning needed for this "mild to wild" dish.

1 pound chicken tenders or tenderloins, all visible fat removed

Vegetable oil spray

3 cups frozen chopped mixed bell
peppers and onions, thawed

14.5-ounce can no-salt-added diced
tomatoes, drained

1 cup spicy-style Bloody Mary mix or
low-sodium spicy mixed-vegetable
juice

½ teaspoon dried thyme, crumbled, or
to taste

½ teaspoon red hot-pepper sauce, or
to taste

2¼ cups uncooked instant rice

¼ cup snipped fresh parsley

2 teaspoons extra-virgin olive oil

(PER SERVING)

Calories 318

Protein 24 g

Carbohydrates 43 g

Cholesterol 53 mg

Total Fat 4 g

  Saturated 1 g

  Polyunsaturated 1 g

  Monounsaturated 2 g

Fiber 3 g

Sodium 356 mg

Rinse chicken and pat dry with paper towels. If using tenderloins, cut each into three or four strips.

Heat a large nonstick skillet over medium-high heat for 1 minute. Remove from heat and spray with vegetable oil spray. Cook chicken for 4 minutes, stirring occasionally; set aside on a plate.

Away from heat, spray skillet again with vegetable oil spray. Cook peppers and onions for 2 minutes, or until onions are translucent, stirring frequently.

Add tomatoes, Bloody Mary mix, thyme, hot-pepper sauce, and chicken with any accumulated juices; bring to a boil. Reduce heat and simmer, uncovered, for 10 minutes, stirring occasionally.

Meanwhile, cook rice using package directions, omitting salt and oil.

Remove chicken mixture from heat. Stir in parsley and oil; let stand, uncovered, for 2 to 5 minutes.

To serve, arrange rice on serving platter; spoon chicken mixture over rice.

POULTRY

Dilled Chicken with Mushrooms and Rice

Serves 4; 1¾ cups per serving ∎
Preparation time: 10 minutes ∎
Cooking time: 28 minutes ∎

Here's a comforting chicken and rice dish for your repertoire, and this one has only a single pan to wash.

Vegetable oil spray

1½ cups chopped onion (yellow preferred) (3 medium)

1 pound chicken tenders or tenderloins, all visible fat removed

8 ounces presliced fresh mushrooms

2 cups water

1 cup uncooked rice

1 tablespoon dried dillweed, crumbled

¼ to ½ teaspoon salt

2 tablespoons lemon juice

¼ teaspoon salt

2 teaspoons extra-virgin olive oil

Paprika (optional)

Heat a 12-inch nonstick skillet or Dutch oven over medium-high heat. Remove from heat and spray with vegetable oil spray. Add onions and cook for 5 minutes, or until translucent, stirring frequently.

Meanwhile, rinse chicken and pat dry with paper towels. If using tenderloins, cut into strips about ½ inch wide.

Add chicken, mushrooms, water, rice, dillweed, and ½ teaspoon salt to onions, stirring well; bring to a boil. Reduce heat and simmer, covered, for 20 minutes, or until water is absorbed and rice is tender. Remove from heat.

Stir in lemon juice and ¼ teaspoon salt.

Drizzle with olive oil, then sprinkle lightly with paprika.

(PER SERVING)

Calories 358

Protein 30 g

Carbohydrates 46 g

Cholesterol 66 mg

Total Fat 6 g

   Saturated 1 g

   Polyunsaturated 1 g

   Monounsaturated 3 g

Fiber 3 g

Sodium 411 mg

Bell Pepper Chicken and Noodles

- Serves 5; 1½ cups per serving
- Preparation time: 15 minutes
- Cooking time: 18 minutes

Although this dish is delicious if served immediately, the chicken and noodles absorb even more flavors if the mixture has time to sit for a while.

12 ounces chicken tenders or tenderloins, all visible fat removed

1 cup reduced-sodium chicken broth

¼ cup no-salt-added ketchup

1 teaspoon dried oregano, crumbled

½ teaspoon salt

Vegetable oil spray

3 cups frozen chopped green bell pepper; 2 large green bell peppers, thinly sliced (about 12 ounces); or 1 large green bell pepper and 2 poblano chiles, thinly sliced

2 cups frozen chopped onion or 1 large onion, thinly sliced (yellow preferred) (about 8 ounces)

14.5-ounce can no-salt-added diced tomatoes

4 ounces dried no-yolk egg noodles

1 tablespoon plus 1 teaspoon no-salt-added ketchup

¼ teaspoon salt

(PER SERVING)

Calories 222

Protein 21 g

Carbohydrates 29 g

Cholesterol 39 mg

Total Fat 2 g

  Saturated 1 g

  Polyunsaturated 1 g

  Monounsaturated 1 g

Fiber 3 g

Sodium 425 mg

Rinse chicken and pat dry with paper towels; set aside.

In a small bowl, whisk together broth, ¼ cup ketchup, oregano, and ½ teaspoon salt until well blended; set aside.

Heat a Dutch oven over medium-high heat until very hot. Remove from heat and spray with vegetable oil spray. Cook chicken for 3 minutes, stirring frequently.

Increase heat to high. Add peppers, onion, undrained tomatoes, noodles, and broth mixture; bring to a boil. Reduce heat and simmer, covered, for 13 minutes, stirring occasionally. Remove from heat.

Stir in remaining ingredients.

Chicken Fajita Pasta
with Chipotle Alfredo Sauce

Serves 5; 1½ cups per serving ■
Preparation time: 10 minutes ■
Cooking time: 25 to 30 minutes ■

Buy marinated chicken fajita meat at the grocery store, choosing the one with the lowest sodium, or marinate chicken tenders in a low-sodium fajita marinade. You can even use leftover cooked chicken or lean beef. Warm it with the pasta and the sauce.

8 ounces dried rigatoni

8 ounces uncooked marinated chicken fajita meat, all visible fat removed

1 teaspoon olive oil

¾ cup frozen chopped onion or 1 large onion, thinly sliced

2 cups frozen bell pepper strips or 1 large green bell pepper and 1 large red bell pepper, thinly sliced

¾ cup fat-free evaporated milk

1 teaspoon bottled chipotle sauce

⅛ teaspoon pepper

1 medium yellow tomato, cut into 8 wedges (optional)

¼ cup sliced black olives (optional)

Prepare rigatoni using package directions, omitting salt and oil. Drain, return to pan off heat, and set aside.

Meanwhile, thinly slice chicken; set aside.

Heat a large nonstick skillet over medium-high heat. Add oil and swirl to coat bottom of skillet. Cook onion and bell peppers for 2 to 3 minutes, or until tender, stirring occasionally. Push to one side of skillet.

Add chicken and cook for 6 to 8 minutes, or until no longer pink in center, stirring occasionally. (When chicken is browned, stir onion mixture in and cook together until chicken is done.)

Meanwhile, in a measuring cup or small bowl, combine milk, chipotle sauce, and pepper.

Add chicken and milk mixture to cooked pasta. Cook over low heat for 1 to 2 minutes, or until warmed, stirring occasionally.

To serve, garnish with tomato and olives.

(PER SERVING)

Calories 266

Protein 19 g

Carbohydrates 43 g

Cholesterol 21 mg

Total Fat 3 g

  Saturated 1 g

  Polyunsaturated 0 g

  Monounsaturated 1 g

Fiber 2 g

Sodium 272 mg

Greek Chicken Thighs

- Serves 6; 2 ounces chicken and ½ cup bulgur mixture per serving
- Preparation time: 5 minutes
- Cooking time: 35 to 37 minutes

You'll think you're at a taverna on the Mediterranean Sea when you bite into these chicken thighs. They're packed with flavor from lemon, feta cheese, oregano, and Greek olives.

6 boneless, skinless chicken thighs, all visible fat removed (about 1 pound)

Olive oil spray

1 cup low-sodium chicken broth

1 cup water

1 teaspoon dried oregano, crumbled

1 teaspoon lemon zest

2 teaspoons lemon juice

⅛ teaspoon pepper

1 cup uncooked bulgur wheat

8 Greek olives, pitted (about 1 ounce)

2 tablespoons feta cheese, rinsed and crumbled

Rinse chicken and pat dry with paper towels.

Heat a large, deep skillet or Dutch oven over medium-high heat. Remove from heat and spray with olive oil spray. Return to heat and cook chicken for 3 minutes on each side.

Add broth, water, oregano, lemon zest, lemon juice, and pepper to skillet. Bring to a simmer over medium-high heat, about 2 minutes. Reduce heat to medium-low and cook, covered, for 15 minutes, or until chicken is no longer pink in center. Remove chicken.

Stir remaining ingredients into skillet; return chicken to skillet. Cook, covered, over medium-low heat for 10 minutes, or until bulgur is tender.

(PER SERVING)

Calories 237

Protein 18 g

Carbohydrates 23 g

Cholesterol 52 mg

Total Fat 8 g

Saturated 2 g

Polyunsaturated 1 g

Monounsaturated 2 g

Fiber 3 g

Sodium 168 mg

Polynesian Chicken in a Slow Cooker

Serves 6; ⅔ cup per serving ■
Preparation time: 5 minutes ■
Cooking time: 8 to 9 hours ■

Because they're moister and more flavorful, chicken thighs are better than white meat for long cooking. The pineapple juice provides a subtle sweetness to this dish, which goes well over steamed rice.

Vegetable oil spray

1½ pounds boneless, skinless chicken thighs or 2 pounds chicken thighs, skinned, all visible fat removed

⅔ cup pineapple juice (6-ounce can)

3 tablespoons vinegar

3 tablespoons light soy sauce

1 tablespoon grated gingerroot

¼ teaspoon crushed red pepper flakes

Spray a 3½- to 4-quart slow cooker with vegetable oil spray.

Rinse chicken and pat dry with paper towels. Put in slow cooker and add remaining ingredients. Cook on low for 8 to 9 hours.

MEDITERRANEAN CHICKEN IN A SLOW COOKER

Substitute 14.5-ounce can no-salt-added crushed or diced tomatoes, undrained, for the pineapple juice; substitute 1 teaspoon dried oregano, crumbled, and 1 teaspoon bottled minced garlic or 2 medium cloves, minced, for the gingerroot. Serve over no-yolk noodles instead of rice. (Calories 178; Protein 20 g; Carbohydrates 4 g; Cholesterol 70 mg; Total Fat 8 g; Saturated 2 g; Polyunsaturated 2 g; Monounsaturated 3 g; Fiber 1 g; Sodium 266 mg)

(PER SERVING)

Calories 177

Protein 20 g

Carbohydrates 5 g

Cholesterol 70 mg

Total Fat 8 g

   Saturated 2 g

    Polyunsaturated 2 g

    Monounsaturated 3 g

Fiber 0 g

Sodium 260 mg

Southwestern-Style Roasted Chicken

- Serves 9; 3 ounces chicken per serving (plus 12 ounces reserved)
- Preparation time: 10 minutes
- Cooking time: 3 hours
- Standing time: 15 minutes

What's an almost-3½-hour recipe doing in a quick and easy cookbook? Well, for 3¼ hours, you don't need to lift a finger. Plus, you get plenty of chicken for Sunday dinner and for later in the week, perhaps in Sour Cream Chicken Enchiladas (page 170).

7-pound roasting chicken, giblets removed

1 medium lime, quartered

2 medium shallots or ½ small onion, halved

1 teaspoon cumin seeds or ground cumin

3 or 4 sprigs fresh cilantro

2 tablespoons lime juice (1 to 2 medium limes)

1 teaspoon chili powder

1 teaspoon ground cumin

1 teaspoon dried oregano, crumbled

Vegetable oil spray

Preheat oven to 350° F.

Rinse chicken and pat dry with paper towels. Put chicken on a rack in a shallow roasting pan.

Put lime, shallots, cumin, and cilantro in chicken cavity, then pour lime juice over chicken.

In a small bowl, stir together chili powder, ground cumin, and oregano. Rub into skin of chicken.

Tie chicken legs together with kitchen twine. Lightly spray chicken with vegetable oil spray.

Bake, uncovered, for about 3 hours. If chicken starts to get too brown, put a piece of aluminum foil loosely over top. Chicken is done when juices run clear from a thigh pierced with a fork or when a meat thermometer inserted between thigh and breast registers 180° F (make sure thermometer is not touching bone).

Let chicken stand for 15 minutes before carving. Remove and discard skin before serving chicken.

Cook's Tip on Chicken Yield

A 7-pound roasting chicken yields about:
   18 ounces breast meat
    8 ounces thigh meat
    6 ounces leg meat
    4 ounces wing meat
    3 ounces back meat

As a rule of thumb, figure that boneless, skinless chicken will lose about one fourth of its weight when cooked. Therefore, a boneless, skinless breast that weighs 4 ounces raw will weigh about 3 ounces cooked.

Time-Saver

Disposable plastic gloves are an inexpensive time-saver. Use them when rubbing an herb or spice mixture on poultry, as in this recipe, or when handling meat or seafood. Keep in mind that you should still wash your hands after removing the gloves, but because your hands will be much cleaner to start with, the washing up will be quicker.

(PER SERVING)
Calories 171
Protein 25 g
Carbohydrates 1 g
Cholesterol 77 mg
Total Fat 7 g
   Saturated 2 g
    Polyunsaturated 1 g
    Monounsaturated 2 g
Fiber 0 g
Sodium 78 mg

Sour Cream Chicken Enchiladas

- Serves 6; 2 enchiladas per serving
- Preparation time: 20 minutes
- Cooking time: 19 to 22 minutes

Create this mouthwatering favorite with the leftover chicken from Southwestern-Style Roasted Chicken (pages 168–169) or other cooked chicken. Serve with pinto beans and slaw.

Sauce

1¼ cups low-sodium chicken broth

1 tablespoon plus 1 teaspoon cornstarch

½ teaspoon ground cumin

⅛ teaspoon black pepper

■ ■ ■

12 6-inch corn tortillas

12 ounces cooked skinless chicken breast, chopped (about 3 cups)

4 ounces fat-free or low-fat cream cheese

½ cup salsa

Vegetable oil spray

¾ cup nonfat or light sour cream

2 teaspoons lime juice

¼ teaspoon chili powder (optional)

In a small saucepan, whisk together sauce ingredients. Bring to a simmer over medium-high heat and cook for 1 to 2 minutes, or until mixture is thick and bubbly; set aside.

Put tortillas in a tortilla warmer or wrap them in damp paper towels and microwave on high for 30 to 60 seconds.

Preheat oven to 350° F.

In a medium nonstick skillet, combine chicken, cream cheese, and salsa. Cook over medium-low heat for 5 to 6 minutes, or until mixture is warmed through and cream cheese has melted, stirring occasionally.

Lightly spray a 13 x 9 x 2-inch baking dish with vegetable oil spray.

To assemble, pour ½ cup sauce into baking dish; spread to cover bottom of dish. Put a tortilla on a plate or cutting board. Spoon about ¼ cup chicken mixture onto middle of tortilla. Roll tortilla jelly-roll style and place seam side down in baking dish. Repeat with remaining tortillas and filling. Pour remaining sauce over enchiladas. Cover dish with aluminum foil.

Bake for 10 minutes, or until filling is warmed through.

Meanwhile, in a small bowl, whisk together sour cream and lime juice. When enchiladas have baked for 10 minutes, spread mixture on top. Bake, uncovered, for about 2 minutes, or until topping is slightly warm. Sprinkle with chili powder.

COOK'S TIP

If you don't have a microwave, you can warm the tortillas in the oven. Wrap the tortillas in aluminum foil. When you turn on the oven, put the tortillas in the preheating oven for at least 5 minutes, or until soft and pliable.

TIME-SAVER

For a quick casserole, preheat oven to 350° F. Cut or tear tortillas in half. Put them on an ungreased baking sheet and bake for 5 minutes, or until slightly crisp on the edges and somewhat soft in the center. Spread ½ cup sauce in the prepared baking dish. Layer half the tortillas over the sauce. Spread the chicken mixture over the tortillas. Layer the remaining tortillas over the chicken mixture; top with remaining sauce. Bake as directed.

(PER SERVING)

Calories 296
Protein 26 g
Carbohydrates 38 g
Cholesterol 55 mg
Total Fat 4 g
    Saturated 1 g
    Polyunsaturated 1 g
    Monounsaturated 1 g
Fiber 4 g
Sodium 395 mg

Curried Chicken, Pasta, and Vegetable Casserole

- Serves 5; 1½ cups per serving
- Preparation time: 10 minutes
- Cooking time: 23 to 26 minutes
- Standing time: 5 to 10 minutes

What could be easier than cooking the pasta with the other ingredients, all at one time and all in one pot?

2¼ cups fat-free milk

10-ounce can reduced-fat cream of chicken soup

1-pound bag frozen mixed broccoli, mushrooms, onions, and green beans

6 ounces dried rotini (about 2½ cups)

2 cups diced cooked skinless chicken breast (3 to 4 ounces)

½ to ¾ teaspoon curry powder

⅛ teaspoon cayenne (optional)

In a large bowl, whisk together milk and soup. Pour into a 3-quart saucepan or 12-inch nonstick skillet. Bring just to a boil over medium-high heat, about 10 minutes, stirring frequently with a rubber scraper.

Stir in vegetables and pasta; return to a boil. Reduce heat and simmer, uncovered, for 12 to 15 minutes, or until pasta is tender, stirring frequently. Remove from heat.

Stir in remaining ingredients. Let stand, uncovered, for 5 to 10 minutes to absorb flavors and thicken slightly.

CURRIED PASTA AND VEGETABLE CASSEROLE

For a vegetarian variation, omit the chicken and substitute reduced-fat cream of mushroom soup for the cream of chicken soup. Serves 4; 1½ cups per serving. (Calories 282; Protein 12 g; Carbohydrates 52 g; Cholesterol 8 mg; Total Fat 2 g; Saturated 1 g; Polyunsaturated 1 g; Monounsaturated 0 g; Fiber 26 g; Sodium 419 mg)

Chicken, Pasta, and Vegetable Casserole

Substitute frozen mixed broccoli, cauliflower, and red bell peppers for broccoli, mushrooms, onions, and green beans; dried spaghetti, broken in half, for rotini; and a 2-ounce jar of chopped pimientos, drained, for curry powder. After cooking, top with 2 ounces shredded reduced-fat sharp Cheddar cheese. The cheese will melt during the standing time. Serves 5; 1½ cups per serving. (Calories 347; Protein 33 g; Carbohydrates 41 g; Cholesterol 62 mg; Total Fat 6 g; Saturated 2 g; Polyunsaturated 1 g; Monounsaturated 2 g; Fiber 3 g; Sodium 457 mg)

Pasta and Vegetable Casserole

To turn the Chicken, Pasta, and Vegetable Casserole into a vegetarian entrée, omit the chicken and substitute reduced-fat cream of mushroom soup for cream of chicken soup. Serves 4; 1½ cups per serving. (Calories 314; Protein 18 g; Carbohydrates 51 g; Cholesterol 18 mg; Total Fat 5 g; Saturated 2 g; Polyunsaturated 1 g; Monounsaturated 1 g; Fiber 4 g; Sodium 506 mg)

(PER SERVING)

Calories 321

Protein 28 g

Carbohydrates 42 g

Cholesterol 55 mg

Total Fat 4 g

  Saturated 1 g

  Polyunsaturated 1 g

  Monounsaturated 1 g

Fiber 21 g

Sodium 388 mg

Lemongrass Chicken with Snow Peas and Jasmine Rice

- Serves 4; 1 cup chicken mixture and ½ cup rice per serving
- Preparation time: 5 minutes
- Cooking time: 20 to 25 minutes

Transform leftover cooked chicken into a dish that will delight the senses with color, texture, aroma, and flavor. Lemongrass, Thai red chili paste, and coconut (our heart-healthy recipe uses coconut extract) are the popular Thai ingredients that do the trick.

¾ cup uncooked jasmine rice

1½ cups water

1 stalk lemongrass or 1 teaspoon lemon zest

2 cups low-sodium chicken broth

2 cups water

2 cups diced cooked skinless chicken breast (3 to 4 ounces)

1 cup snow peas, cut into thin strips (about 3 ounces)

2 green onions, thinly sliced (about ¼ cup)

1 tablespoon Thai red curry sauce

½ teaspoon coconut extract

(PER SERVING)

Calories 314

Protein 25 g

Carbohydrates 33 g

Cholesterol 63 mg

Total Fat 8 g

　Saturated 1 g

　Polyunsaturated —

　Monounsaturated —

Fiber 2 g

Sodium 405 mg

Cook rice using package directions except use 1½ cups water and omit salt and margarine.

Meanwhile, trim about 6 inches off slender tip end of lemongrass stalk and discard. Remove outer layer of leaves from bottom part of stalk. Carefully cut stalk in half lengthwise. Put in a large saucepan.

Add broth, 2 cups water, and chicken to pan; bring to a boil over high heat. Reduce heat to medium-low and cook, covered, for 6 to 8 minutes, or until mixture has a lemon flavor; don't stir. Remove lemongrass and discard.

Add remaining ingredients (if you are using lemon zest instead of lemongrass, add it now). Cook for 1 to 2 minutes, or until snow peas are tender-crisp, stirring occasionally.

To serve, put ½ cup rice into each bowl. Top each serving with 1 cup chicken mixture.

Creamed Chicken and Vegetables

Serves 4; 1 cup per serving ■
Preparation time: 5 minutes ■
Cooking time: 20 minutes ■

This simple dish is as pleasing to the eyes as it is to the palate. Savor it as is or over toast or rice.

3 cups frozen mixed peas, carrots, baby corn, and snow peas or mixed peas and carrots

8 ounces frozen cooked diced chicken breast

10-ounce can reduced-fat cream of chicken soup

½ cup canned mushrooms, rinsed and drained

⅓ cup water or low-sodium chicken broth

½ teaspoon dried tarragon, crumbled

¼ teaspoon freshly ground pepper

In a medium saucepan, combine all ingredients. Cook, covered, over medium heat for 20 minutes, or until vegetables are tender and mixture is thoroughly heated, stirring occasionally.

CREAMED TUNA AND VEGETABLES

Substitute two 6-ounce cans tuna packed in spring or distilled water, rinsed and drained, for chicken. (Calories 159; Protein 20 g; Carbohydrates 12 g; Cholesterol 37 mg; Total Fat 3 g; Saturated 1 g; Polyunsaturated 1 g; Monounsaturated 1 g; Fiber 1 g; Sodium 371 mg)

(PER SERVING)

Calories 128

Protein 16 g

Carbohydrates 12 g

Cholesterol 39 mg

Total Fat 2 g

   Saturated 1 g

   Polyunsaturated 0 g

   Monounsaturated 0 g

Fiber 1 g

Sodium 465 mg

Turkey and Broccoli Stir-Fry

- Serves 4; 1 cup per serving
- Preparation time: 15 minutes
- Cooking time: 12 minutes

Both the turkey supper and the vegetarian version are good over long-grain white rice. Add a cup of soup or a fruit salad to round out the meal.

2 tablespoons light soy sauce

1 tablespoon dry sherry

¾ pound turkey scallopine (thinly sliced turkey breast) or boneless, skinless chicken breast halves

Freshly ground pepper

3 tablespoons lemon juice

¼ cup water

1 tablespoon sugar

1 tablespoon light soy sauce

1 tablespoon cornstarch

1 tablespoon bottled minced garlic or 6 medium cloves garlic, minced

1 tablespoon minced gingerroot

2 green onions, minced (green and white parts)

1 fresh jalapeño, seeded and minced, or crushed red pepper flakes, to taste (optional)

1 tablespoon acceptable vegetable oil (divided use)

3 to 4 cups broccoli florets (about 1 pound florets or 2 medium heads)

¼ cup water (plus more as needed)

In a medium bowl, combine 2 tablespoons soy sauce and sherry.

Rinse turkey and pat dry with paper towels. Cut turkey across short side into slivers about ¼ inch wide and 2 inches long. Stir into soy sauce mixture; season with pepper; set aside.

In a small bowl, whisk together lemon juice, ¼ cup water, sugar, and 1 tablespoon soy sauce. Whisk in cornstarch; set aside.

In another small bowl, stir together garlic, gingerroot, green onions, and jalapeño.

Heat a 12-inch skillet, preferably cast iron, a wok, or a Dutch oven over high heat for a full minute. Add 1½ teaspoons oil and swirl to coat bottom of skillet. Stir in half the turkey. Cook for 2 minutes, or until turkey starts becoming opaque, stirring constantly. Transfer to serving bowl and repeat with remaining oil and turkey, plus any remaining marinade.

Stir garlic mixture, broccoli, and ¼ cup water into skillet. Cook, covered, for 3 minutes.

Stir lemon juice mixture to disperse cornstarch. Stir mixture and turkey into skillet. Cook until glossy, 1 to 2 minutes, stirring constantly. Stir in more water to thin sauce if necessary.

VEGETARIAN STIR-FRY

Omit 2 tablespoons light soy sauce, sherry, turkey, and pepper. Beat egg substitute equivalent to 2 eggs, or 2 large eggs, with ¼ teaspoon salt. Chop 4 green onions (green and white parts). Heat skillet over high heat. Add 1 tablespoon vegetable oil. Cook green onions for a few seconds, stirring constantly. Add egg mixture. Cook until softly set (no stirring needed); remove to plate. Continue as directed above, replacing turkey with egg mixture. Serves 4; ¾ to 1 cup per serving. (Calories 106; Protein 6 g; Carbohydrates 13 g; Cholesterol 0 mg; Total Fat 4 g; Saturated 0 g; Polyunsaturated 2 g; Monounsaturated 1 g; Fiber 3 g; Sodium 319 mg)

COOK'S TIP

You can substitute boneless, skinless chicken breasts cut into slivers for the turkey in this recipe. Preparation goes faster if you buy the broccoli florets at your supermarket salad bar.

COOK'S TIP ON STIR-FRYING

Old-fashioned cast-iron skillets are excellent for stir-frying. Black metal absorbs heat well, and the iron will hold onto the heat after you add the meat and vegetables. Unlike woks, which may teeter on American stoves (woks actually are made to sit in wells), skillets sit flat and drink up all the heat and Btu's a U.S. stove can crank out.

(PER SERVING)

Calories 191
Protein 23 g
Carbohydrates 14 g
Cholesterol 55 mg
Total Fat 5 g
  Saturated 1 g
  Polyunsaturated 2 g
  Monounsaturated 1 g
Fiber 3 g
Sodium 352 mg

Turkey Cutlets with Two Sauces

- Serves 4; 3 ounces turkey, 1 cup spaghetti squash, and ¼ cup sauce per serving
- Preparation time: 5 minutes
- Cooking time: 43 to 45 minutes

Can't decide whether you prefer spaghetti sauce or Alfredo sauce? With this double-sauced casserole, you get to enjoy both.

Olive oil spray

4 cups cooked spaghetti squash or spaghetti (about 2½ pounds uncooked squash or 8 ounces uncooked spaghetti)

½ cup low-sodium chicken broth (¾ cup if using spaghetti)

1 pound turkey cutlets or strips, all visible fat removed

¼ cup plain dry bread crumbs

½ cup fat-free meatless spaghetti sauce

½ cup light Alfredo sauce

Preheat oven to 375° F. Spray a 1½-quart shallow baking dish or 13 x 9 x 2-inch baking dish with olive oil spray.

Spread squash in dish; pour broth over squash.

Rinse turkey and pat dry with paper towels. Place turkey in one layer over squash.

Sprinkle turkey with bread crumbs and lightly spray with olive oil spray. Cover baking dish tightly with aluminum foil.

Bake for 35 minutes. Pour spaghetti sauce and Alfredo sauce over casserole. Bake, uncovered, for 8 to 10 minutes, or until sauce is warmed through and turkey is no longer pink in center.

COOK'S TIP ON SPAGHETTI SQUASH

To bake spaghetti squash, preheat oven to 350° F. Put a 2½-pound spaghetti squash on a baking sheet. Prick the squash several times with a fork. Bake, uncovered, for 45 to 50 minutes, or until squash feels slightly tender when squeezed (use an oven mitt for this). Cut the squash in half lengthwise. Let squash cool for about 5 minutes. Remove seeds with a spoon. With a fork, scrape the spaghetti-like squash strands from the shell into a bowl. Serve as is, or top with your favorite low-fat sauce.

To microwave, place the spaghetti squash in a glass pie plate and prick. Microwave on 100 percent power (high), uncovered, for 15 to 20 minutes, or until squash feels tender when squeezed.

To steam, cut the spaghetti squash in half lengthwise and remove seeds. Cut each piece in half. Place squash in a steamer basket in a medium saucepan over simmering water. Cook, covered, for 15 to 20 minutes, or until tender.

Cooked squash will keep in an airtight container for up to five days in the refrigerator. A 2½-pound spaghetti squash yields about 4 cups of cooked "spaghetti."

(PER SERVING)

Calories 268
Protein 28 g
Carbohydrates 20 g
Cholesterol 89 mg
Total Fat 8 g
  Saturated 4 g
  Polyunsaturated 1 g
  Monounsaturated 2 g
Fiber 3 g
Sodium 454 mg

Italian Bean Stew with Turkey and Ham

- Serves 4; 2 cups per serving
- Preparation time: 5 minutes
- Cooking time: 18 to 19 minutes

This bubbling stew incorporates the basics of a traditional Italian dish called ribollita but takes much less time. A savory way to use leftover ham, it's just right for warming up a small crowd before the Friday-night football game.

1 tablespoon olive oil

1 pound ground skinless turkey breast

1 teaspoon fennel seeds, crushed if desired (optional)

2 15-ounce cans no-salt-added navy beans, rinsed and drained

3 cups low-sodium chicken broth

9-ounce package frozen no-salt-added Italian green beans (1½ cups)

1 cup diced low-fat, lower-sodium ham (4 ounces)

1 teaspoon bottled minced garlic or 2 medium cloves garlic, minced

½ teaspoon dried thyme, crumbled

½ teaspoon dried oregano, crumbled

¼ teaspoon pepper

Heat a Dutch oven over medium-high heat. Add oil and swirl to coat bottom of pot. Cook turkey and fennel seeds for 6 to 8 minutes, or until turkey is no longer pink, stirring occasionally.

Add remaining ingredients and bring to a boil over high heat. Reduce heat to medium-low and cook, covered, for 10 minutes, or until green beans are tender, stirring occasionally. Serve at once or continue cooking for up to 1 hour.

(PER SERVING)

Calories 454

Protein 51 g

Carbohydrates 46 g

Cholesterol 77 mg

Total Fat 9 g

  Saturated 2 g

  Polyunsaturated 1 g

  Monounsaturated 3 g

Fiber 2 g

Sodium 412 mg

Grilled Turkey Cutlets with Pineapple

Serves 4; 3 ounces turkey and 1 pineapple ring per serving ■
Preparation time: 10 minutes ■
Marinating time: 10 minutes to 8 hours ■
Cooking time: 8 to 10 minutes ■

Serve these citrus-flavored cutlets with sweet potatoes sprinkled with nutmeg, or put a cutlet and a pineapple slice in a bun and enjoy as a sandwich. Double the recipe except the pineapple slices and use the extra turkey for Turkey Tortilla Soup (page 56).

2 tablespoons lime juice (1 to 2 medium limes)

1 tablespoon orange-flavored liqueur or orange juice

2 teaspoons acceptable vegetable oil

½ teaspoon dried oregano, crumbled

¼ teaspoon pepper

1 pound skinless turkey breast, all visible fat removed

4 slices pineapple canned in their own juice

In a large airtight plastic bag, combine lime juice, liqueur, oil, oregano, and pepper.

Rinse turkey and pat dry with paper towels. Slice turkey into cutlets ½ inch thick. Add to marinade, turning to coat. Refrigerate for 10 minutes to 8 hours. Turn occasionally if marinating more than 10 minutes.

Preheat grill on medium-high.

Grill turkey for 4 to 5 minutes on each side, or until no longer pink in center, turning once (no need to drain marinade). Transfer to a serving platter.

Grill pineapple slices for 1 minute on each side. Place on turkey.

COOK'S TIP ON TURKEY CUTLETS

To make cutlets from a turkey breast, use a sharp knife and slice the turkey at a slight angle into ½-inch cutlets.

(PER SERVING)

Calories 172

Protein 27 g

Carbohydrates 8 g

Cholesterol 73 mg

Total Fat 3 g

  Saturated 1 g

  Polyunsaturated 2 g

  Monounsaturated 1 g

Fiber 1 g

Sodium 47 mg

Turkey Breast with Cranberry Sage Stuffing

- Serves 6; 3 ounces turkey and ¼ cup gravy per serving
- Preparation time: 15 minutes
- Cooking time: 55 minutes to 1 hour

You may want to prepare this meal quite often—not just for company—when you see how easy it is. Use leftover slices in our Cranberry and Cream Cheese Turkey Sandwiches on page 102.

Stuffing

1 rib celery, diced (about ½ cup)

1 leek (white part only) or ½ small onion, diced

½ 6-inch whole-wheat pita, torn into small pieces

½ cup dried cranberries

¼ cup low-sodium chicken broth

1 teaspoon rubbed or crumbled sage

⅛ teaspoon pepper

■ ■ ■

1½-pound boneless, skinless turkey breast, all visible fat removed

1 tablespoon acceptable vegetable oil

2 cups low-sodium chicken broth

½ cup water

¼ cup all-purpose flour

In a medium bowl, combine all stuffing ingredients.

Rinse turkey and pat dry with paper towels. Butterfly turkey by cutting it lengthwise down the center, *almost* in half; don't cut completely through. Lay out flat and lightly cover with plastic wrap. Using flat side of a meat mallet, pound turkey to flatten slightly. (Perhaps your butcher will do this for you.)

Place stuffing down middle of turkey. Roll turkey around stuffing and tie at 2-inch intervals with kitchen twine.

Preheat oven to 350° F.

Heat a Dutch oven over medium-high heat. Add oil and swirl to coat bottom of pot. Brown turkey for 2 minutes on each side.

Pour 2 cups broth over turkey.

Bake, covered, for 45 to 50 minutes, or until turkey is no longer pink and internal temperature reaches 170° F. Transfer turkey to a carving board; set aside.

Bring liquid in Dutch oven to a boil over medium-high heat.

Meanwhile, in a small bowl, whisk together water and flour. Whisk into boiling broth mixture and cook for 3 to 4 minutes, or until gravy is thick and bubbly.

To serve, ladle ¼ cup gravy onto each of six plates. Place 1 slice turkey on each serving of gravy.

COOK'S TIP ON MESH

Kitchen twine is a great way to secure roasts and help them keep their shape while cooking. Butchers use a similar product that is stringlike, is stretchy, and, with a bit of maneuvering, can easily cover a roast. Many butchers will sell—or perhaps even give—you a small amount of mesh to use at home. For large quantities, check restaurant supply or specialty stores.

(PER SERVING)

Calories 233

Protein 29 g

Carbohydrates 19 g

Cholesterol 74 mg

Total Fat 4 g

Saturated 1 g

Polyunsaturated 2 g

Monounsaturated 1 g

Fiber 2 g

Sodium 130 mg

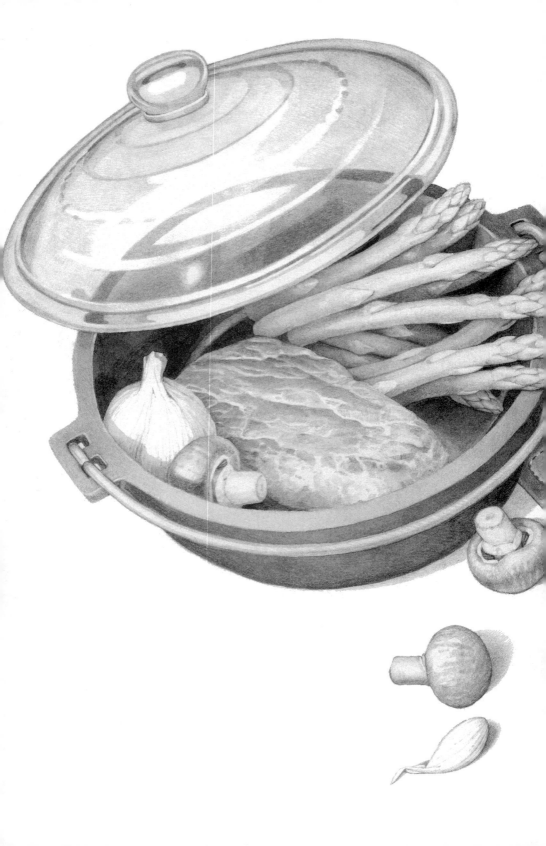

MEATS

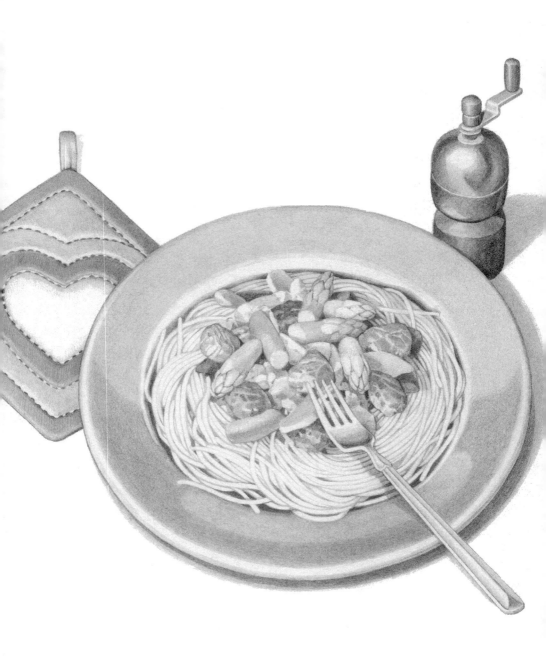

■ ■ ■

Grilled Sirloin with Honey
Mustard Marinade

Glazed Beef Strips
with Sugar Snap Peas

Burgundy Beef Stew

Beef with Rice Noodles
and Vegetables

Beef Strips with Caramelized
Onions and Mashed Potatoes

Taco-Rubbed Flank Steak

Beef Tenderloin
with Mixed Baby Greens

Tuscan Braised Beef

Roast Beef with Baby Carrots,
Onions, and Potatoes

Blue Cheese Beef and Fries

Chili-Style Beef Stew

Picante Meat Loaf
with Baked Potatoes

Tex-Mex Rice and Meatballs

Ground Beef and Shredded
Potato Casserole

Beef with Barley and Vegetables

No-Chop Stew

Mediterranean Beef and Rice

Cheddar Jack Chili Mac

Cajun Skillet Supper

Parmesan Pork Medallions

Roasted Lemon Pork with
Cinnamon Sweet Potatoes

Orange Sesame Pork

Red-Hot Pork Stir-Fry

Red-Hot Chicken Stir-Fry

Cook's-Choice Fried Rice

Asian Pork Stir-Fry

Rosemary Braised Pork Chops

Celery-Sage Pork Chops

Blackberry-Glazed Pork
with Mixed Rice and Broccoli

Ham and Vegetable Casserole

Sweet-and-Sour Black-Eyed Peas
with Ham

Ham and Hash Brown Casserole

Smoked Sausage Skillet Supper

Curried Lamb Stew
with Chick-Peas

French Veal Stew

French Turkey Stew

■ ■ ■

Grilled Sirloin with Honey Mustard Marinade

Serves 4; 3 ounces meat per serving (plus 12 ounces reserved) ■
Preparation time: 10 minutes ■
Marinating time: 24 to 48 hours ■
Cooking time: 15 minutes ■

This steak is ideal for entertaining outdoors, and you get a bonus—enough meat to make another meal, such as Beef and Caramelized Onion on Hot French Bread.

2 pounds boneless top sirloin steak, all visible fat removed

Marinade

⅓ cup prepared mustard

¼ cup honey

1 to 2 teaspoons crushed red pepper flakes

1 teaspoon cider vinegar

Put steak in a large airtight plastic bag.

In a small bowl, whisk together marinade ingredients until well blended. Refrigerate ¼ cup marinade. Pour remaining marinade over steak, seal bag, and turn to coat. Refrigerate for 24 to 48 hours, turning occasionally.

Preheat grill and grill rack on medium-high.

Drain steak, discarding marinade in bag. Cook steak, covered, for 5 minutes. Turn over, baste with 2 tablespoons reserved marinade, and cook for 5 minutes. Turn over, baste with remaining marinade, and cook for 5 minutes, or until desired doneness. Cut diagonally into strips, reserving half (about 12 ounces) for Beef and Caramelized Onion on Hot French Bread (page 104).

Cook's Tip

Freeze the steak and marinade in the plastic bag. The freezing and thawing time is the marinating time.

(PER SERVING)

Calories 173

Protein 22 g

Carbohydrates 2 g

Cholesterol 64 mg

Total Fat 6 g

　Saturated 2 g

　Polyunsaturated 0 g

　Monounsaturated 2 g

Fiber 0 g

Sodium 109 mg

Glazed Beef Strips with Sugar Snap Peas

- Serves 4; 1 cup per serving
- Preparation time: 20 minutes
- Marinating time: 10 minutes to 12 hours
- Cooking time: 11 to 14 minutes

This recipe boasts a Japanese marinade and a slightly sweet glaze. Like many other Asian stir-fries, it goes well over steamed rice.

1 pound boneless sirloin, all visible fat removed

Marinade

¼ cup chopped frozen onion, ½ medium onion, chopped, or 2 green onions, thinly sliced

2 tablespoons sake or dry white wine (regular or nonalcoholic)

1 teaspoon wasabi powder (optional)

¼ teaspoon ground ginger or 1 teaspoon grated gingerroot

1 teaspoon light soy sauce

Glaze

¼ cup low-sodium beef broth

1 tablespoon plus 1½ teaspoons light brown sugar

1 tablespoon low-sodium teriyaki sauce

■ ■ ■

2 cups fresh or frozen sugar snap peas (8 ounces)

Vegetable oil spray

1 teaspoon sesame seeds (optional)

Cut beef into thin strips.

In a medium bowl, stir together marinade ingredients. Stir in beef strips and cover bowl with plastic wrap; set aside for 10 minutes or refrigerate for up to 12 hours.

For glaze, stir together all ingredients in a small bowl; set aside.

If using fresh peas, trim ends; set peas aside.

Heat a large nonstick skillet over medium-high heat. Remove from heat and lightly spray with vegetable oil spray. Cook meat with any remaining marinade for 3 to 4 minutes, or until browned, stirring occasionally.

Add glaze and cook for 6 to 7 minutes. Add peas and cook for 1 to 2 minutes, or until most liquid is gone and meat is glazed, stirring occasionally. Sprinkle with sesame seeds.

COOK'S TIP ON WASABI

Also known as Japanese horseradish, wasabi is available in paste and powder. Both pack a powerful pungency, so add wasabi in small amounts. The powder form of this light green condiment is usually mixed with water or other liquids.

(PER SERVING)

Calories 198

Protein 25 g

Carbohydrates 10 g

Cholesterol 64 mg

Total Fat 6 g

    Saturated 2 g

    Polyunsaturated 0 g

    Monounsaturated 2 g

Fiber 2 g

Sodium 175 mg

Burgundy Beef Stew

- Serves 9; 1 cup per serving
- Preparation time: 20 minutes
- Cooking time: 37 minutes
- Standing time: 10 minutes

An almost-effortless dish, this stew requires no peeling and little or no cutting!

2 cups water

6-ounce can no-salt-added tomato paste (¾ cup)

1-ounce package dried onion soup mix

2 tablespoons dry red wine (regular or nonalcoholic) (optional)

1½ teaspoons light soy sauce

2 teaspoons dried oregano, crumbled

½ teaspoon sugar

Vegetable oil spray

16 ounces boneless sirloin, all visible fat removed, cut into 1-inch pieces

16-ounce bag frozen stew vegetables

2 cups frozen chopped green bell peppers

10-ounce package frozen no-salt-added cut green beans

Pepper to taste

(PER SERVING)

Calories 212

Protein 12 g

Carbohydrates 15 g

Cholesterol 28 mg

Total Fat 3 g

  Saturated 1 g

  Polyunsaturated 0 g

  Monounsaturated 1 g

Fiber 3 g

Sodium 370 mg

In a medium bowl, whisk together water, tomato paste, soup mix, wine, soy sauce, oregano, and sugar; set aside.

Heat a Dutch oven over high heat until very hot. Remove from heat and spray with vegetable oil spray. Brown meat for 2 to 3 minutes, stirring frequently.

Stir in remaining ingredients, including tomato paste mixture; bring to a boil. Reduce heat and simmer, covered, for 30 minutes, stirring occasionally. Remove from heat.

Cut potatoes in half. Stir stew, then sprinkle with pepper. Cover and let stand for 10 minutes to allow flavors to blend.

TIME-SAVER

To save time and energy, ask your butcher to trim and cut the beef while you finish shopping.

Beef with Rice Noodles and Vegetables

Serves 6; 1¼ cups per serving ■
Preparation time: 15 minutes ■
Cooking time: 8 minutes ■

Chunks of beef are browned and simmered in this tasty Asian stew.

1 teaspoon acceptable vegetable oil

1 pound boneless sirloin or beef tenderloin, all visible fat removed, cut into ¾-inch cubes

2 cups presliced fresh mushrooms (about 8 ounces)

1 medium carrot, cut into thin strips

1 teaspoon bottled minced garlic or 2 medium cloves garlic, minced

2 cups low-sodium beef broth

1 cup asparagus pieces about ½ inch long

1 tablespoon light soy sauce

¼ teaspoon chili oil

2 ounces rice noodles or dried angel hair pasta

6 ounces frozen no-salt-added collard greens or leaf spinach or about 1 pound fresh collard greens or spinach, very thinly sliced

½ teaspoon toasted sesame oil

1 lime, cut into wedges or wheels (optional)

Heat a Dutch oven over medium-high heat. Add oil and swirl to cover bottom of pot. Cook meat for 2 minutes, or until brown, stirring occasionally.

Add mushrooms, carrot, and garlic; cook for 1 minute, stirring occasionally.

Add broth, asparagus, soy sauce, and chili oil; bring to a boil over high heat, 1 to 2 minutes.

Add remaining ingredients except lime. Cook, covered, over low heat for 5 minutes, or until noodles are tender. Use tongs to transfer noodles to bowls. Ladle broth and vegetables into bowls. Serve with lime.

COOK'S TIP ON RICE NOODLES

Find thin rice noodles, sometimes called rice-flavor noodles, in the Asian section of your grocery store.

(PER SERVING)

Calories 171

Protein 18 g

Carbohydrates 14 g

Cholesterol 43 mg

Total Fat 5 g

  Saturated 1 g

  Polyunsaturated 1 g

  Monounsaturated 2 g

Fiber 2 g

Sodium 183 mg

Beef Strips with Caramelized Onions and Mashed Potatoes

- Serves 4; 1 cup meat mixture and ½ cup mashed potatoes per serving
- Preparation time: 10 minutes
- Cooking time: 26 to 32 minutes

The timesaving secret to this recipe is to start cooking the onions first. Another time-saver: Use leftover mashed potatoes, premashed potatoes (from the refrigerated section of your grocery), or instant mashed potatoes.

1 teaspoon olive oil

1 teaspoon acceptable margarine

1 large onion, thinly sliced

Olive oil spray

1 pound boneless beef round steak, all visible fat removed, cut into thin strips

1 cup low-sodium beef broth

½ cup dry white wine (regular or nonalcoholic) or low-sodium beef broth

1 teaspoon bottled minced garlic or 2 medium cloves garlic, minced

2 cups mashed potatoes (about 1 pound raw)

3 tablespoons water

2 tablespoons all-purpose flour

(PER SERVING)

Calories 300

Protein 25 g

Carbohydrates 26 g

Cholesterol 64 mg

Total Fat 8 g

  Saturated 2 g

  Polyunsaturated 1 g

  Monounsaturated 4 g

Fiber 3 g

Sodium 97 mg

Heat a large skillet over medium heat. Add oil, margarine, and onions; cook, covered, for 2 minutes, or until onions are soft. Increase heat to medium-high and cook, uncovered, for 20 to 25 minutes, or until onions are golden brown, stirring occasionally.

Meanwhile, heat a large skillet (preferably *not* nonstick) over medium-high heat. Remove from heat and spray with olive oil spray. Cook beef for 5 to 6 minutes, stirring occasionally.

Add broth, wine, and garlic; bring to a simmer over medium-high heat. Reduce heat to medium-low and cook, covered, until onions are ready. (Meat will become tenderer the longer it cooks.)

Heat or prepare mashed potatoes.

Meanwhile, in a small bowl, whisk together water and flour. Add with onions to beef. Cook over medium-high heat until mixture is thick and bubbly, 3 to 4 minutes.

To serve, spoon ½ cup mashed potatoes onto each plate and spoon meat mixture over potatoes.

Taco-Rubbed Flank Steak

Serves 6; 3 ounces meat per serving (plus 6 ounces reserved) ■
Preparation time: 10 minutes ■
Cooking time: 10 to 30 minutes ■

To add lots of flavor and no fat to meats, rub it in with a spice rub. Make the rub from mild to extra-spicy, depending on the level of heat you like best. Use leftovers from this recipe for Flank Steak Burritos.

Rub

2 tablespoons chili powder

2 teaspoons ground cumin

1 teaspoon dried oregano, crumbled

¼ to 1 teaspoon cayenne

½ teaspoon salt

½ teaspoon sugar

■ ■ ■

1 medium lime

2 pounds flank steak, all visible fat removed

Preheat grill on high or preheat broiler.

For rub, combine all ingredients in a small bowl.

Squeeze lime over steak and rub juice into meat. Rub with chili powder mixture to coat completely.

Grill steak or broil 5 to 6 inches from heat until desired doneness (about 5 minutes on each side for medium-rare to 15 minutes per side for well-done). Reserve 6 ounces (about one fourth) for Flank Steak Burritos (page 103).

COOK'S TIP ON GRILLING OR BROILING

Timing your grilling or broiling can be tricky. Different grills and broilers give off different amounts of heat, and the distance from the heat affects how quickly the meat cooks, as does whether the meat is chilled. Of course, the thickness of the cut also makes a difference. Watch your meat, and cut into the center to check for doneness.

(PER SERVING)

Calories 119

Protein 15 g

Carbohydrates 2 g

Cholesterol 36 mg

Total Fat 6 g

  Saturated 2 g

  Polyunsaturated 0 g

  Monounsaturated 2 g

Fiber 1 g

Sodium 156 mg

Beef Tenderloin with Mixed Baby Greens

- Serves 4; 3 ounces meat and 1 cup mixed baby greens per serving
- Preparation time: 15 minutes
- Cooking time: 25 to 27 minutes

A quick sauce of broth and balsamic vinegar picks up the tantalizing flavor of the caramelized brown bits left in the cooking pan. The sauce tops a stack of baby greens, garlic toast, and sliced beef—an elegant presentation worthy of company.

Garlic Toasts

4 slices French bread, about ¾-inch thick (4 ounces)

Olive oil spray

1 teaspoon bottled minced garlic or 2 medium cloves garlic, minced

Sauce

½ cup low-sodium beef broth

½ cup water

¼ cup balsamic vinegar

2 tablespoons light brown sugar

¼ teaspoon pepper

■ ■ ■

4 cups mixed baby greens or baby spinach leaves (about 5 ounces)

1-pound beef tenderloin, all visible fat removed

1 teaspoon olive oil

Preheat oven to 375° F.

For garlic toasts, put bread slices on a small ungreased baking sheet. Lightly spray both sides of bread with olive oil spray. Spread about ¼ teaspoon garlic over each slice.

Bake for 10 minutes, or until bread is toasted and lightly golden. Let cool on a cooling rack; set aside. (Garlic toasts can be prepared ahead and refrigerated for up to three days in an airtight container.)

While the bread is toasting, whisk together sauce ingredients in a small bowl; set aside.

Line up four dinner plates. Arrange 1 cup salad greens on each plate, mounding slightly in center. Place a garlic toast gently in center of each mound.

Slice meat crosswise into 4 pieces.

Heat a large skillet (preferably *not* nonstick) over medium-high heat. Add oil and swirl to coat bottom of skillet. Cook meat for 5 minutes. Turn meat over (a flexible metal spatula works best) and cook for 4 to 6 minutes, or until meat reaches desired doneness (5 minutes per side for medium-rare to medium). Carefully place each piece of meat on top of a slice of garlic toast.

Immediately add sauce mixture to skillet. With a wooden spoon, scrape and loosen brown bits on bottom of skillet. Cook over high heat without stirring for 5 minutes, or until mixture is reduced by half.

Just before serving, pour about 2 tablespoons sauce over each serving of beef and greens.

COOK'S TIP ON DEGLAZING

The secret to many a great sauce is those crunchy bits left in the pan after the meat or vegetables are browned. To incorporate their rich, caramelized flavor into the sauce, deglaze the pan: Add a liquid and reduce the sauce either by boiling it at a high temperature without stirring or by thickening it with a mixture such as flour or cornstarch and water. A nonstick pan is not a good choice when making sauces and gravies by deglazing because no brown bits will stick to it.

(PER SERVING)

Calories 298

Protein 25 g

Carbohydrates 27 g

Cholesterol 61 mg

Total Fat 10 g

  Saturated 3 g

  Polyunsaturated 0 g

  Monounsaturated 4 g

Fiber 2 g

Sodium 274 mg

Tuscan Braised Beef

- Serves 4; 3 ounces meat and ¼ cup gravy per serving (plus 12 ounces reserved)
- Preparation time: 10 minutes
- Cooking time: 2½ to 3 hours *or*
  Slow-cooker time: 4 to 5 hours on high or 8 to 10 hours on low
- Standing time: 10 to 15 minutes (both methods)

A taste of Italy, this tender roast gets a robust herb rub and then is left to bake. It's great for Sunday dinner, or start it in the slow cooker before you go to work. Among the recipes we've included for using the planned-over portion are Beef Salad with Vinaigrette or Horseradish Dressing, Thai Beef Salad, and Blue Cheese Beef and Fries (pages 86–87, 88, and 200).

Rub

1 tablespoon dried rosemary, crushed

2 teaspoons bottled minced roasted or plain garlic or 4 medium cloves garlic, minced

1 teaspoon dried ground or rubbed sage

1 teaspoon grated lemon zest

¼ teaspoon salt

¼ teaspoon pepper

■ ■ ■

2 pounds eye-of-round roast, all visible fat removed

2 cups low-sodium beef broth

⅓ cup water

3 tablespoons all-purpose flour

Preheat oven to 350° F.

In a small bowl, stir together rub ingredients. Using a pastry brush or your hands, brush or rub mixture over roast. Put roast in an ungreased Dutch oven; pour broth around roast.

Cover Dutch oven with aluminum foil; put lid over foil. (See Cook's Tip on Lean Meat, page 199.) Bake for 2½ to 3 hours, or until roast is tender or registers an internal temperature of 140° F to 150° F (for medium) on a meat or instant-read thermometer. Transfer to a carving board, reserving liquid. Cover roast with aluminum foil and let stand for 10 to 15 minutes before carving.

Bring reserved liquid to a simmer over medium-high heat.

Meanwhile, in a small bowl, whisk together water and flour. Whisk mixture into simmering broth. Cook for 2 to 3 minutes, or until thick and bubbly, whisking occasionally.

To serve, pour gravy over roast.

Slow-Cooker Method

Apply rub mixture to roast as directed. Put roast in a 3½- to 4-quart slow cooker and pour in beef broth. Cover and cook on high for 4 to 5 hours or on low for 8 to 10 hours, or until roast is tender. When roast is done, remove from cooker and let stand as directed. To make gravy, pour liquid from cooker into a medium saucepan and thicken with flour mixture as directed.

COOK'S TIP ON INSTANT-READ THERMOMETERS

When you insert an instant-read thermometer's long, thin metal probe into food, the tool instantly lets you know the food's internal temperature. Don't insert this kind of thermometer into the food and then bake it; the thermometer may melt. Meat thermometers, on the other hand, are made to stay in food while cooking.

Eye-of-round roast is cooked to the medium stage when the thermometer reads 140° F to 150° F, medium-well when the internal temperature is 155° F to 165° F, and well-done between 170° F and 185° F.

(PER SERVING)

Calories 163

Protein 25 g

Carbohydrates 3 g

Cholesterol 57 mg

Total Fat 5 g

   Saturated 2 g

   Polyunsaturated 0 g

   Monounsaturated 2 g

Fiber 0 g

Sodium 163 mg

Roast Beef with Baby Carrots, Onions, and Potatoes

- Serves 4; 3 ounces meat and ¼ cup vegetables per serving (plus 12 ounces meat and 3 cups vegetables reserved)
- Preparation time: 20 minutes
- Cooking time: 1 hour 15 minutes
- Standing time: 10 minutes

While the roast and vegetables cook, you'll have plenty of time to prepare and chill Peach Fans on Blackberry-Lime Sauce (page 74) for a combination of salad and dessert. Using the entrée leftovers later in the week, you can make a second, totally different dish—Chili-Style Beef Stew.

Vegetable oil spray

2 pounds eye-of-round roast, all visible fat removed

16 ounces very small red potatoes (about 16 1-ounce potatoes)

2 medium onions, cut into eighths (yellow preferred) (about 10 ounces)

12 ounces baby carrots (about 1½ cups)

¼ cup dry red wine (regular or nonalcoholic) or low-sodium beef broth

1 tablespoon bottled minced roasted or plain garlic or 6 medium cloves garlic, minced

1½ to 2 teaspoons salt-free lemon pepper

1 teaspoon paprika

2 teaspoons water

1 teaspoon very low sodium or low-sodium Worcestershire sauce

1 tablespoon all-purpose flour

Preheat oven to 325° F.

Heat a Dutch oven over high heat until very hot. Remove from heat and heavily spray with vegetable oil spray. Return to heat and sear beef on one side for about 45 seconds; don't let meat burn. Turn meat over. Remove Dutch oven from heat.

Put vegetables, wine, and garlic around meat; sprinkle all with lemon pepper and paprika.

Cover Dutch oven with aluminum foil; put lid over foil. Bake for 1 hour and 5 minutes, or until internal temperature of meat registers 155° F on a meat or instant-read thermometer.

Put meat on cutting board and let stand for 10 minutes. Cut meat in half, reserving one piece (about ¼ pound) and half the vegetables (about 3 cups) for Chili-Style Beef Stew (page 201).

Cut remaining meat into 8 slices and place on serving platter. Arrange remaining 3 cups vegetables around meat. Cover with aluminum foil to keep warm.

In a small bowl, whisk together remaining ingredients until well blended.

Bring pan drippings to a boil over high heat. Whisk in flour mixture. Boil for 2 to 5 minutes, or until gravy thickens and measures about ¼ cup, whisking constantly. Spoon over meat.

Cook's Tip

If you can't find 1-ounce potatoes, cut larger red potatoes into halves or quarters, depending on size.

Cook's Tip on Lean Meat

Sometimes lean cuts of meat, such as eye-of-round roast, can become dry while cooking. To keep this from happening, cover your pot with aluminum foil, then with the lid.

(PER SERVING)

Calories 240
Protein 26 g
Carbohydrates 20 g
Cholesterol 57 mg
Total Fat 5 g
    Saturated 2 g
    Polyunsaturated 0 g
    Monounsaturated 2 g
Fiber 3 g
Sodium 73 mg

Blue Cheese Beef and Fries

- Serves 4; 1¼ cups per serving
- Preparation time: 10 minutes
- Cooking time: 31 to 32 minutes

Top oven fries with the works—tender beef, brown gravy, and a bit of blue cheese for a zesty flavor. You can use leftover roast beef, such as the extra Tuscan Braised Beef (pages 196–197), or buy the lowest-fat, lowest-sodium cooked beef you can find.

Olive oil spray

4 medium red potatoes, cut into ⅛- to ¼-inch strips (about 1⅓ pounds)

½ teaspoon garlic powder

½ teaspoon paprika

⅛ teaspoon pepper

2 cups thinly sliced cooked roast beef, all visible fat removed (about 8 ounces)

2 cups frozen broccoli florets, thawed

1 cup fat-free brown gravy

1 tablespoon plus 1 teaspoon crumbled blue cheese

Preheat oven to 400° F. Spray a nonstick jelly-roll pan with olive oil spray. Arrange potatoes evenly in pan.

In a cup, combine garlic powder, paprika, and pepper. Sprinkle over potatoes.

Bake for 25 minutes, or until potatoes are tender.

Put beef and broccoli on potatoes. Top with gravy.

Bake for 6 to 7 minutes, or until mixture is warmed through. Sprinkle with cheese.

(PER SERVING)

Calories 254

Protein 22 g

Carbohydrates 34 g

Cholesterol 48 mg

Total Fat 4 g

  Saturated 2 g

  Polyunsaturated 0 g

  Monounsaturated 2 g

Fiber 4 g

Sodium 440 mg

COOK'S TIP ON FAT-FREE GRAVY

Look in the sauces section of your grocery store for bottles of fat-free brown (or beef) and chicken gravy.

COOK'S TIP

A mandoline makes fast work of slicing. Use the very fine julienne blade to cut the potatoes into matchstick size for this recipe. A food processor with a French-fry blade is equally good.

Chili-Style Beef Stew

Serves 4; 1½ cups per serving ■
Preparation time: 10 minutes ■
Cooking time: 35 minutes ■

Starting with planned-overs from Roast Beef with Baby Carrots, Onions, and Potatoes makes easy work of preparing this dish, which has the slow-roasted flavors of a campfire stew. Stirring in part of the cumin at serving time gives the stew a more pronounced chili flavor.

12 ounces roast reserved from Roast Beef with Baby Carrots, Onions, and Potatoes (pages 198–199)

3 cups vegetables reserved from Roast Beef with Baby Carrots, Onions, and Potatoes

15-ounce can no-salt-added dark kidney beans, rinsed and drained

14.5-ounce can no-salt-added diced tomatoes

½ cup water

2 teaspoons ground cumin

2 tablespoons no-salt-added ketchup or 1 tablespoon no-salt-added tomato paste and 1½ teaspoons sugar

1 teaspoon ground cumin

Cut beef and potatoes into bite-size pieces. Put in a Dutch oven and stir in onions, carrots, beans, undrained tomatoes, water, and 2 teaspoons cumin; cover and bring to a boil over high heat. Reduce heat and simmer, covered, for 25 minutes.

Remove from heat and stir in remaining ingredients.

(PER SERVING)

Calories 371

Protein 33 g

Carbohydrates 44 g

Cholesterol 57 mg

Total Fat 6 g

   Saturated 2 g

    Polyunsaturated 1 g

    Monounsaturated 2 g

Fiber 10 g

Sodium 91 mg

Picante Meat Loaf with Baked Potatoes

- Serves 4; 3 ounces meat loaf and 1 potato per serving
- Preparation time: 15 minutes
- Cooking time: 1 hour

Blend lean ground beef with salsa and chopped peppers for the ultimate dish after an exhausting day. All you do is mix, mold, and relax! Green beans or mixed vegetables would round out the meal nicely.

Vegetable oil spray

Meat Loaf

1 pound lean ground beef

1 cup frozen chopped green bell pepper or mixed bell pepper strips, or 1 large green bell pepper, chopped or thinly sliced

¼ cup rolled oats

½ cup picante sauce

White of 1 large egg

1 teaspoon very low sodium or low-sodium Worcestershire sauce

■ ■ ■

2 tablespoons no-salt-added ketchup

¼ teaspoon very low sodium or low-sodium Worcestershire sauce

4 6-ounce red potatoes

Preheat oven to 350° F. Spray a broiler pan and rack or a roasting pan and baking rack with vegetable oil spray.

In a medium bowl, combine meat loaf ingredients. Shape into a 5 x 7-inch oval loaf and place on rack.

Combine ketchup and ¼ teaspoon Worcestershire sauce. Spread evenly over top and sides of meat loaf. Place rack in baking pan.

Arrange potatoes on rack around meat loaf.

Bake for 1 hour, or until meat is no longer pink in center and potatoes are tender.

(PER SERVING)

Calories 370

Protein 27 g

Carbohydrates 44 g

Cholesterol 70 mg

Total Fat 10 g

Saturated 4 g

Polyunsaturated 1 g

Monounsaturated 4 g

Fiber 4 g

Sodium 232 mg

Tex-Mex Rice and Meatballs

Serves 4; 6 meatballs and ½ cup rice per serving ■
Preparation time: 10 minutes ■
Cooking time: 25 minutes ■

If you're a fan of spaghetti and meatballs, try our Tex-Mex variation on that theme. Serve your favorite low-sodium salsa on the side for those who want more heat.

14.5-ounce can no-salt-added tomatoes, slightly crushed

1 cup water

⅔ cup uncooked rice

1 teaspoon ground cumin

½ to 1 teaspoon chili powder

¼ teaspoon salt

Vegetable oil spray

1 pound lean ground beef

2 6-inch corn tortillas, diced

Egg substitute equivalent to 1 egg, or 1 large egg

1 teaspoon chili powder

½ teaspoon onion powder

½ teaspoon garlic powder

½ teaspoon ground cumin

¼ teaspoon salt

In a medium saucepan, bring tomatoes and water to a boil over high heat.

Stir in rice, 1 teaspoon cumin, ½ to 1 teaspoon chili powder, and ¼ teaspoon salt. Reduce heat and simmer, covered, for 20 minutes, or until rice is tender.

Meanwhile, preheat broiler. Spray a broiler pan and rack with vegetable oil spray.

In a medium bowl, combine remaining ingredients, using your hands to mix. Using a rounded tablespoon measure, shape into 24 meatballs (about 1-inch diameter) and place on broiler rack.

Leave oven door slightly ajar and broil meatballs about 6 inches from heat for 4 minutes, or until brown on top. Turn meatballs over. Broil for 2 to 4 minutes, or until no longer pink in center, watching carefully to keep meatballs from burning.

To serve, spoon rice onto serving plate and place meatballs on top.

(PER SERVING)

Calories 384

Protein 34 g

Carbohydrates 38 g

Cholesterol 70 mg

Total Fat 10 g

Saturated 4 g

Polyunsaturated —

Monounsaturated —

Fiber 3 g

Sodium 448 mg

Ground Beef and Shredded Potato Casserole

- Serves 4; 1¼ cups per serving
- Preparation time: 10 minutes
- Cooking time: 25 minutes

When the family wants meat and potatoes, this flexible recipe will come to mind. Almost any quick-cooking frozen vegetable or combination works well in it.

Vegetable oil spray

8-ounce can no-salt-added tomato sauce (1 cup)

¼ teaspoon sugar (optional)

1 pound lean ground beef

1 teaspoon salt-free all-purpose seasoning

½ to ¾ teaspoon dried basil, dried oregano, or combination, crumbled

½ teaspoon ground cumin

¼ teaspoon salt

⅛ teaspoon pepper

1 teaspoon bottled minced garlic or 2 medium cloves garlic, minced

½ to ¾ cup frozen chopped onion or 1 medium to large onion, chopped

1 cup frozen no-salt-added corn, carrots, or green beans; frozen peas; or combination

2 cups frozen nonfat shredded hash brown potatoes

¼ cup water

Preheat oven to 450° F. Spray a shallow 1½-quart baking dish with vegetable oil spray.

In a small bowl, stir together tomato sauce and sugar; set aside.

Using your hands, break apart beef into ½- to 1-inch pieces (irregular pieces are okay); layer in baking dish, leaving slight space between pieces.

Sprinkle beef with all-purpose seasoning, basil, cumin, salt, and pepper.

Top with garlic, onions, tomato sauce mixture, frozen vegetables, and potatoes. Pour water over all. Lightly spray potatoes with vegetable oil spray.

Bake, covered, for 25 minutes, or until pieces of beef are no longer pink in center and potatoes are tender.

COOK'S TIP

If time allows, prepare the recipe as directed through topping the ground beef with the seasonings, onions, and tomato sauce mixture. Cover the baking dish and refrigerate for 10 to 30 minutes to let flavors permeate the meat. Add the remaining ingredients as directed. Put the dish in a cold oven, set the oven to 450° F, and bake for 35 to 40 minutes.

(PER SERVING)

Calories 231

Protein 24 g

Carbohydrates 14 g

Cholesterol 70 mg

Total Fat 9 g

   Saturated 4 g

    Polyunsaturated 0 g

    Monounsaturated 4 g

Fiber 2 g

Sodium 235 mg

Beef with Barley and Vegetables

- Serves 4; 1½ cups per serving
- Preparation time: 5 minutes
- Cooking time: 26 to 30 minutes

This hearty one-dish meal is a tummy-warming choice meant for a chilly evening.

1 pound lean ground beef

2 medium potatoes, cut into 1-inch cubes (10 ounces)

1 cup low-sodium beef broth

1 cup water

1 teaspoon onion powder

1 teaspoon garlic powder

½ teaspoon dried thyme, crumbled

¼ teaspoon salt

⅛ teaspoon pepper

15-ounce can sweet potatoes, drained

2 cups frozen no-salt-added green beans

¼ cup quick-cooking barley

Heat a Dutch oven over medium-high heat. Cook ground beef for 8 to 10 minutes, or until no longer pink, stirring occasionally. Put beef in a colander and rinse with hot water to remove excess fat; drain well. Wipe Dutch oven clean with paper towel. Return beef to Dutch oven.

Add potatoes, broth, water, onion powder, garlic powder, thyme, salt, and pepper. Bring to a boil over high heat. Reduce heat to medium-low and cook, covered, for 8 to 10 minutes, or until potatoes are tender.

Stir in remaining ingredients and cook over medium-low heat for 10 minutes, or until barley is tender.

COOK'S TIP

If you stir as little as possible, the potatoes hold their shape better.

COOK'S TIP ON QUICK-COOKING BARLEY

Look for quick-cooking barley in the supermarket's hot cereal section. If you can't find it, you can use regular barley instead. Add it with the potatoes and cook for 20 to 30 minutes instead of 10 in the final step.

(PER SERVING)

Calories 364

Protein 33 g

Carbohydrates 44 g

Cholesterol 70 mg

Total Fat 7 g

  Saturated 3 g

  Polyunsaturated 1 g

  Monounsaturated 3 g

Fiber 6 g

Sodium 272 mg

No-Chop Stew

Serves 6; 1½ cups per serving ■
Preparation time: 10 minutes ■
Cooking time: 34 to 36 minutes ■
❶

This hefty dinner in a bowl is a great comfort after a hectic day, especially since you don't need to chop anything to prepare it.

1 pound lean ground beef

2 14.5-ounce cans no-salt-added diced or stewed tomatoes

3 cups shredded coleslaw mix (about 6 ounces)

2 cups water

10-ounce package frozen mixed vegetables, thawed

1 cup frozen chopped green bell pepper or 1 large green bell pepper, chopped

¼ cup cider vinegar or dry red wine (regular or nonalcoholic)

1 tablespoon reduced-sodium beef bouillon granules

1 tablespoon dried oregano, crumbled

½ teaspoon sugar

¼ cup finely snipped fresh parsley

1 teaspoon salt

Pepper to taste

Heat a Dutch oven over high heat. Cook beef until brown, 3 to 4 minutes, stirring frequently. Put beef in a colander and rinse with hot water to remove excess fat; drain well. Wipe pot with paper towel; return beef.

Add undrained tomatoes, coleslaw, water, mixed vegetables, bell pepper, vinegar, bouillon, oregano, and sugar to beef; bring to a boil over high heat. Reduce heat and simmer, covered, for 30 minutes. Remove from heat.

Stir in parsley, salt, and pepper.

COOK'S TIP

This is a great make-ahead dish, and it freezes well too.

(PER SERVING)

Calories 198

Protein 22 g

Carbohydrates 18 g

Cholesterol 47 mg

Total Fat 5 g

  Saturated 2 g

  Polyunsaturated 1 g

  Monounsaturated 2 g

Fiber 6 g

Sodium 399 mg

Mediterranean Beef and Rice

- Serves 6; 1¼ cups per serving
- Preparation time: 5 minutes
- Cooking time: 22 to 23 minutes

When you need a satisfying meal that uses ground beef, try this recipe. It's as easy as 1-2-3. Just brown the beef, heat the sauce, and add the rice. Then ring the dinner bell!

1 pound lean ground beef

14.5-ounce can no-salt-added stewed tomatoes

1 cup water

1 teaspoon dried oregano, crumbled

1 teaspoon garlic powder

½ teaspoon paprika

½ teaspoon salt-free lemon pepper

½ teaspoon salt

15-ounce can no-salt-added navy beans, rinsed and drained

15-ounce can no-salt-added French-style green beans, drained

1 cup uncooked instant brown rice

In a large skillet, cook beef over medium-high heat for 7 to 8 minutes, or until browned on outside and no longer pink in center, stirring occasionally. Put beef in a colander and rinse with hot water to remove excess fat; drain well. Wipe skillet with paper towels. Return beef to skillet.

Stir in tomatoes, water, oregano, garlic powder, paprika, lemon pepper, and salt. Cook, uncovered, over medium heat for 5 minutes, stirring occasionally.

Stir in remaining ingredients and cook, covered, over medium-low heat for 5 minutes. Turn off heat and let stand for 5 minutes, or until rice is tender.

(PER SERVING)

Calories 275

Protein 25 g

Carbohydrates 34 g

Cholesterol 47 mg

Total Fat 5 g

  Saturated 2 g

  Polyunsaturated 0 g

  Monounsaturated 2 g

Fiber 3 g

Sodium 266 mg

Cheddar Jack Chili Mac

Serves 5; 1½ cups per serving ■
Preparation time: 5 minutes ■
Cooking time: 19 to 25 minutes ■

A classic dish gets a quick makeover. Some flavor combinations never go out of style!

1 pound lean ground beef

3 cups water

15-ounce can no-salt-added stewed tomatoes

8-ounce can no-salt-added tomato sauce (1 cup)

1 teaspoon bottled minced garlic or 2 medium cloves garlic, minced

1 teaspoon dried oregano, crumbled

½ teaspoon sugar

½ teaspoon salt

⅛ teaspoon pepper

1 cup dried macaroni or other small pasta

¼ cup fat-free or reduced-fat shredded Cheddar or Monterey Jack cheese or a combination (about 1 ounce)

In a Dutch oven, cook beef over medium-high heat for 8 to 10 minutes, or until no longer pink, stirring occasionally. Put beef in a colander and rinse with hot water to remove excess fat; drain well. Wipe Dutch oven with a paper towel; return beef to pot.

Stir in water, tomatoes, tomato sauce, garlic, oregano, sugar, salt, and pepper. Bring to a boil, covered, over high heat, 1 to 2 minutes.

Stir in macaroni, reduce heat, and simmer for 10 to 12 minutes, or until tender. Ladle mixture into soup bowls. Sprinkle with cheese.

Cook's Tip

Instead of oregano, substitute 1 teaspoon of your favorite spice or dried herb. Here are some suggestions: chili powder, rosemary, ground cumin, thyme, basil, or fennel seeds.

(PER SERVING)

Calories 256

Protein 27 g

Carbohydrates 24 g

Cholesterol 56 mg

Total Fat 6 g

  Saturated 3 g

  Polyunsaturated 0 g

  Monounsaturated 2 g

Fiber 2 g

Sodium 366 mg

Cajun Skillet Supper

- Serves 4; 1½ cups per serving
- Preparation time: 5 minutes
- Cooking time: 13 to 16 minutes

If you like gumbo, you will like this one-dish beef meal. This recipe lends itself well to experimentation, so try different vegetables and beans for variety. To stretch the number of servings, ladle the mixture over steamed rice.

1 pound lean ground beef

2 cups frozen cut okra (unbreaded) (about 16 ounces)

15-ounce can no-salt-added corn, rinsed and drained

15-ounce can no-salt-added kidney beans, rinsed and drained, or 14.25-ounce can no-salt-added stewed tomatoes, undrained

2 cups low-sodium beef broth (1 cup if using stewed tomatoes)

1 teaspoon ground cumin

1 teaspoon chili powder

1 teaspoon dried thyme, crumbled

1 teaspoon garlic powder

1 teaspoon onion powder

⅛ teaspoon pepper

Heat a large nonstick skillet over medium-high heat. Cook beef for 5 to 6 minutes, or until no longer pink, stirring occasionally. Put in a colander and rinse with hot water to remove excess fat; drain well. Wipe skillet with a paper towel.

Return beef to skillet and add remaining ingredients. Bring to a simmer over medium-high heat. Reduce heat and simmer, uncovered, for 8 to 10 minutes, or until flavors are blended, stirring occasionally.

Cook's Tip on Low-Sodium Beef Broth

If you can't find low-sodium beef broth and don't want to make your own, you can use half regular beef broth and half water instead.

(PER SERVING)

Calories 367

Protein 38 g

Carbohydrates 39 g

Cholesterol 70 mg

Total Fat 9 g

  Saturated 3 g

  Polyunsaturated 1 g

  Monounsaturated 3 g

Fiber 8 g

Sodium 160 mg

06/04/2007

Parmesan Pork Medallions

Serves 4; 3 ounces meat and ½ cup asparagus per serving ■
Preparation time: 10 minutes ■
Cooking time: 30 minutes ■

This quick, attractive dish is company-pleasing fare.

Olive oil spray

1 pound pork tenderloin, all visible fat removed

¼ cup all-purpose flour

Egg substitute equivalent to 1 egg, or 1 large egg

½ cup plain dry bread crumbs

½ teaspoon salt-free Italian seasoning

12 ounces fresh asparagus (12 to 15 medium spears)

8-ounce can no-salt-added tomato sauce (1 cup)

1 teaspoon salt-free Italian seasoning

1 tablespoon plus 1½ teaspoons shredded or grated Parmesan cheese

¼ cup crumbled goat cheese

Preheat oven to 400° F. Spray a shallow baking pan with olive oil spray.

Cut pork crosswise into 12 slices. Put with flour in a large airtight plastic bag; shake to coat.

Pour egg substitute into bag and shake to coat.

Combine bread crumbs and ½ teaspoon Italian seasoning in a shallow bowl. Lightly coat pork with bread crumbs. Put pork in baking pan. Lightly spray pork with olive oil spray.

Bake for 25 minutes.

Meanwhile, fill a large skillet with water to a depth of 1 inch. Bring to a boil over high heat.

While water heats, trim and discard bottom 1 inch of asparagus. Add spears to boiling water; reduce heat to medium-high. Cook for 2 to 3 minutes, or until tender-crisp; drain. Cover and set aside.

In a small bowl, stir together tomato sauce and 1 teaspoon Italian seasoning. After pork has baked for 25 minutes, spoon tomato sauce over it. Sprinkle with Parmesan and goat cheese. Bake for 5 minutes, or until pork is no longer pink in center and cheese has melted.

Place asparagus on a platter and top with pork.

(PER SERVING)

Calories 296

Protein 32 g

Carbohydrates 23 g

Cholesterol 74 mg

Total Fat 8 g

Saturated 4 g

Polyunsaturated 1 g

Monounsaturated 3 g

Fiber 3 g

Sodium 282 mg

Roasted Lemon Pork
with Cinnamon Sweet Potatoes

- Serves 4; 3 ounces meat and ½ sweet potato per serving
- Preparation time: 10 minutes
- Cooking time: 55 minutes
- Standing time: 5 minutes

While this meat-and-potatoes combo cooks, prepare a green vegetable and one of our speedy desserts (pages 297–321).

Vegetable oil spray

1-pound pork tenderloin, all visible fat removed

1 medium lemon, cut in half

¼ cup finely snipped fresh parsley

1½ teaspoons bottled minced roasted or plain garlic or 3 medium cloves garlic, minced

½ to 1 teaspoon salt-free lemon pepper

¼ teaspoon salt

2 large sweet potatoes, halved lengthwise (1 to 1½ pounds)

2 teaspoons acceptable margarine, softened

1½ teaspoons dark or light brown sugar

½ teaspoon ground cinnamon

(PER SERVING)

Calories 298

Protein 26 g

Carbohydrates 34 g

Cholesterol 66 mg

Total Fat 7 g

  Saturated 2 g

  Polyunsaturated 1 g

  Monounsaturated 3 g

Fiber 4 g

Sodium 233 mg

Preheat oven to 325° F. Spray broiler pan with vegetable oil spray.

Put pork in pan, tucking any thin ends under to cook evenly. Squeeze lemon over pork, then sprinkle with parsley, garlic, lemon pepper, and salt. Press seasonings onto pork.

Wrap each potato half individually in aluminum foil and place around pork.

Bake for 50 to 55 minutes, or until internal temperature registers 155° F to 160° F on a meat thermometer. (Meat should have a hint of pink. It will cook for a few minutes after you remove it from the oven.)

Meanwhile, in a small bowl, combine remaining ingredients. Stir until smooth; set aside.

When pork is done, remove it from pan and let stand for 5 minutes. (Continue baking potatoes.)

Slice pork and put on platter. Put unwrapped potatoes around pork, and top them with margarine mixture.

Orange Sesame Pork

Serves 4; 3 ounces meat per serving (plus 12 ounces reserved) ■
Preparation time: 10 minutes ■
Cooking time: 20 to 25 minutes ■
Standing time: 5 minutes ■

Toasted sesame seeds add a nuttiness that teams well with pork. You'll be tempted to eat every drop, but save some to make Cook's-Choice Fried Rice (page 216).

1 tablespoon sesame seeds

Vegetable oil spray

2 1-pound pork tenderloins, all visible fat removed

¼ cup rice vinegar, or ¼ cup plain or cider vinegar plus 1 teaspoon sugar

3 tablespoons light soy sauce

2 tablespoons frozen orange juice concentrate or ½ cup orange juice (1 to 2 medium)

2 teaspoons bottled chopped garlic or 4 medium cloves garlic, chopped

⅛ to ¼ teaspoon crushed red pepper flakes

1 to 2 tablespoons water (as needed)

Dry-roast sesame seeds in a small skillet over medium heat for 3 to 4 minutes or in a 375° F oven for 15 minutes, or until golden and aromatic, stirring occasionally.

Meanwhile, preheat oven to 425° F. Spray a 13 x 9 x 2-inch baking pan with vegetable oil spray. Put pork in it so pieces do not touch.

In a small bowl, combine remaining ingredients except water. Pour over pork.

Roast pork for 10 minutes; turn over and roast for 10 to 15 minutes, or until internal temperature registers 155° F to 160° F on a meat or instant-read thermometer. (Meat should have a hint of pink. It will continue to cook for a few minutes after you remove it from oven.) While pork cooks, if sauce appears to be burning (it may burn in corners or in dark pans), tilt pan and loosen and stir thicker sticky substances. Add water if necessary.

Transfer pork to a cutting board and let stand for 5 minutes. Cut diagonally, making long, thin slices.

To serve, sprinkle pork with sesame seeds. Pass pan juices to pour over meat.

(PER SERVING)

Calories 155

Protein 24 g

Carbohydrates 2 g

Cholesterol 66 mg

Total Fat 5 g

   Saturated 1 g

   Polyunsaturated 0 g

   Monounsaturated 2 g

Fiber 0 g

Sodium 193 mg

Red-Hot Pork Stir-Fry

- Serves 4; 1¼ cups per serving
- Preparation time: 12 minutes
- Cooking time: 6 minutes

Here's proof that a home-cooked meal can take less time than making a run for fast food.

1-pound pork tenderloin, all visible
   fat removed
7-ounce box quick-cooking white
   and wild rice
2 tablespoons light soy sauce
2 tablespoons dry sherry
1 tablespoon sugar

½ teaspoon cornstarch
¼ to ½ teaspoon crushed red pepper
   flakes
Vegetable oil spray
1 pound fresh spinach
¼ cup water (divided use)

Cut pork into strips about 2 inches long and ¼ inch wide.

Cook rice using package directions, omitting margarine, salt, and seasoning packet; discard packet.

Meanwhile, in a small bowl, whisk together soy sauce, sherry, sugar, cornstarch, and red pepper flakes until cornstarch is completely dissolved; set aside.

Heat a large nonstick skillet or wok over high heat until very hot. Remove from heat and spray with vegetable oil spray. Cook pork for 3 minutes, stirring constantly.

Add soy sauce mixture and cook until thickened, about 1 minute, stirring constantly. Remove skillet from heat.

Arrange rice on serving platter, leaving room for spinach on outer edge. Spoon pork and sauce over rice; cover with aluminum foil to keep warm.

Return skillet with any pan residue to high heat. Add about half the spinach and 2 tablespoons water. Cook until just limp, about 1 minute, stirring constantly. Arrange around outer edge of rice. Repeat with remaining spinach and water.

Red-Hot Chicken Stir-Fry

Substitute 1 pound boneless, skinless chicken breasts or chicken tenders for pork tenderloin. Rinse and pat dry with paper towels; cut chicken into thin strips. (Calories 346; Protein 33 g; Carbohydrates 44 g; Cholesterol 67 mg; Total Fat 4 g; Saturated 1 g; Polyunsaturated 1 g; Monounsaturated 1 g; Fiber 4 g; Sodium 346 mg)

Cook's Tip

Have your butcher slice the pork for you while you finish shopping, or call ahead so it will be waiting for you—ready when you are and free of charge.

(PER SERVING)
Calories 353
Protein 33 g
Carbohydrates 44 g
Cholesterol 66 mg
Total Fat 5 g
  Saturated 1 g
  Polyunsaturated 1 g
  Monounsaturated 2 g
Fiber 4 g
Sodium 335 mg

Cook's-Choice Fried Rice

- Serves 4; 1½ cups per serving
- Preparation time: 15 minutes
- Cooking time: 12 to 15 minutes

 1

Although this dish calls for leftover Orange Sesame Pork, it's so versatile that you can use almost any leftover meat—from baked chicken to Taco-Rubbed Flank Steak (page 193). No frozen peas and fresh carrots on hand? No problem. Use what you have— bell pepper, broccoli florets, asparagus, or whatever vegetables you prefer. You'll need about 2½ cups in addition to the onion.

1 cup frozen green peas

12 ounces leftover Orange Sesame Pork (page 213) or other cooked meat, cut into ½-inch cubes (about 2 cups)

2 tablespoons light soy sauce

1 tablespoon vinegar (rice vinegar preferred)

2 tablespoons acceptable vegetable oil

2 medium carrots, diced (about 1½ cups)

1 medium onion, sliced (about 1 cup)

¼ teaspoon crushed red pepper flakes

2 cups cooked rice (cold rice preferred)

¼ cup low-sodium chicken broth or water (if using cold rice)

(PER SERVING)

Calories 377

Protein 30 g

Carbohydrates 35 g

Cholesterol 66 mg

Total Fat 12 g

  Saturated 2 g

  Polyunsaturated 5 g

  Monounsaturated 3 g

Fiber 4 g

Sodium 451 mg

Put peas in a colander to begin thawing.

In a medium bowl, stir together pork, soy sauce, and vinegar.

Heat a nonstick wok or large skillet over high heat. Add oil and swirl to coat bottom; heat for about 1 minute, or until very hot. Cook carrots, onion, and red pepper flakes for 4 to 6 minutes, or until vegetables begin to soften, stirring frequently.

Add peas and rice. If using cold rice, add broth. (Hot, moist rice won't need liquid.) Cook for 2 minutes, stirring occasionally to break up rice.

Add pork; stir until it is evenly distributed and all ingredients are heated through, 3 to 5 minutes.

COOK'S TIP ON FRIED RICE

Fried rice is best when made with cold rice, because the rice grains stay firm and separate.

Asian Pork Stir-Fry

Serves 4; 1 cup per serving ■
Preparation time: 10 minutes ■
Cooking time: 11 minutes ■

*Make preparation of this stir-fry easy by getting prewashed spinach from a salad bar.
Serve the finished dish over hot rice.*

1 butterflied pork chop, all visible fat removed (about 6 ounces)

2 tablespoons light soy sauce

1 tablespoon cornstarch

1 teaspoon toasted sesame oil

¼ teaspoon crushed red pepper flakes

1 tablespoon minced gingerroot

1 teaspoon bottled minced garlic or 2 medium cloves garlic, minced

Vegetable oil spray

1 tablespoon plus 1 teaspoon acceptable vegetable oil

8 cups fresh spinach (about 10 ounces or 2 1-quart cartons)

8 ounces presliced fresh mushrooms

2 teaspoons vinegar

2 teaspoons sugar

Cut pork into 1½ x ½-inch strips. Combine in a medium bowl with soy sauce, cornstarch, sesame oil, and red pepper flakes.

Combine ginger and garlic in a small dish.

Heat a nonstick wok or large skillet over high heat. Remove from heat and spray with vegetable oil spray. Cook pork mixture, stirring constantly, until pork is cooked through, about 2 minutes. Remove from wok.

Add vegetable oil to wok and heat for about 30 seconds. Cook gingerroot mixture for about 30 seconds.

Add spinach and mushrooms; cook until spinach is wilted, about 5 minutes, stirring occasionally.

Add pork, vinegar, and sugar. Cook for about 2 minutes, or until heated through, stirring constantly.

COOK'S TIP

Like most stir-fries, this one cooks quickly. That's why you need all the ingredients ready before you heat the wok.

(PER SERVING)

Calories 183

Protein 15 g

Carbohydrates 12 g

Cholesterol 27 mg

Total Fat 10 g

  Saturated 2 g

  Polyunsaturated 3 g

  Monounsaturated 3 g

Fiber 4 g

Sodium 304 mg

Rosemary Braised Pork Chops

- Serves 4; 3 ounces meat per serving
- Preparation time: 5 minutes
- Cooking time: 14 to 19 minutes

No more dry pork chops! Our tender chops are braised to keep them moist. Serve with your favorite green vegetable and Orange-Flavored Acorn Squash and Sweet Potato (page 283).

Rub

1 tablespoon chopped fresh rosemary or 1 teaspoon dried, crushed

1 teaspoon garlic powder

1 teaspoon onion powder

⅛ teaspoon pepper

■ ■ ■

2 butterflied pork chops (about 8 ounces each) or 4 boneless pork loin chops (about 4 ounces each), all visible fat removed (¾ inch thick)

Olive oil spray

½ cup water

In a small bowl, stir together rub ingredients.

Cut pork chops in half if butterflied. Sprinkle both sides with rub.

Heat a large skillet over medium-high heat. Remove from heat and spray with olive oil spray. Put back on heat and cook pork chops for 2 minutes, or until lightly browned. Turn over and cook for 2 minutes.

Add water. Reduce heat to medium-low and cook for 10 to 15 minutes, or until pork is no longer pink in center; drain and serve.

CELERY-SAGE PORK CHOPS

Replace rosemary rub with 1 tablespoon chopped fresh sage (about 10 leaves) or 1 teaspoon dried rubbed or crumbled sage, ½ teaspoon celery seed, ½ teaspoon onion powder, and ⅛ teaspoon pepper.

Cook's Tip

If you have the time or the rest of the meal isn't ready yet, you can simmer these chops for up to 1 hour. (Don't forget to add more water when needed.) Although they'll be fine to eat after 10 to 15 minutes, the pork chops will become even tenderer if cooked longer.

(PER SERVING)

Calories 148

Protein 19 g

Carbohydrates 1 g

Cholesterol 49 mg

Total Fat 7 g

  Saturated 2 g

  Polyunsaturated 1 g

  Monounsaturated 3 g

Fiber 0 g

Sodium 38 mg

Blackberry-Glazed Pork with Mixed Rice and Broccoli

- Serves 4; 3 ounces meat and 1 cup rice mixture per serving
- Preparation time: 15 minutes
- Cooking time: 22 minutes

Sweet, pungent balsamic vinegar provides this richly glazed dish's subtle kick.

½ 6- to 7-ounce box quick-cooking white and wild rice or oriental fried rice, with ½ seasoning packet

2 cups frozen broccoli florets, thawed (8 ounces)

½ cup all-fruit seedless blackberry spread

3 tablespoons balsamic vinegar

Vegetable oil spray

4 4-ounce boneless lean center-cut pork chops, all visible fat removed (about ½ inch thick)

¼ teaspoon dried rosemary, crushed

Cook rice using package directions, omitting salt, margarine, and half the seasoning packet, for 8 minutes. Stir in broccoli; cover and cook for 3 minutes. Remove from heat and set aside, still covered.

Meanwhile, in a small bowl, whisk together jam and vinegar; set aside.

Heat a large nonstick skillet over medium-high heat. Remove from heat and spray with vegetable oil spray. Cook pork for 3 minutes. Turn pork over, sprinkle with rosemary, and cook for 3 minutes, or until lightly browned (pork won't be quite done). Remove from skillet.

Increase heat to high and add blackberry mixture; bring to a boil. Boil for 1 minute; return pork and any juices to skillet. Cook for 1 minute; turn pork over and cook for 45 seconds.

To serve, put rice mixture on serving platter, top with pork, and spoon on remaining glaze.

(PER SERVING)

Calories 336

Protein 24 g

Carbohydrates 46 g

Cholesterol 52 mg

Total Fat 8 g

  Saturated 3 g

  Polyunsaturated 1 g

  Monounsaturated 4 g

Fiber 2 g

Sodium 442 mg

MEATS

Ham and Vegetable Casserole

Serves 5; 1½ cups per serving ■
Preparation time: 15 minutes ■
Cooking time: 18 minutes ■
Standing time: 5 minutes ■

❶

This is a great make-ahead dish because the potatoes absorb lots of flavor as the casserole stands. Just follow the directions in the recipe, but don't add the cheese until right after reheating the dish.

1 pound red potatoes, cut into ⅛-inch slices

2 cups sliced crookneck squash (about 12 ounces)

2 cups frozen chopped green bell pepper (1½ large)

1 cup thinly sliced and chopped low-fat, lower-sodium ham (about 4 ounces)

1 cup frozen chopped onion or 2 medium onions, chopped

¼ cup snipped fresh parsley

2 tablespoons water

¼ teaspoon cayenne

¼ teaspoon salt

3 ounces reduced-fat sharp Cheddar cheese, shredded (about ¾ cup)

Put potatoes, squash, peppers, ham, onions, parsley, water, and cayenne in a Dutch oven; bring to a boil over high heat. Stir to mix thoroughly. Reduce heat and simmer, covered, for 18 minutes, or until potatoes are tender. Remove from heat.

Stir in salt, then sprinkle with cheese. Let stand, uncovered, for 5 minutes to melt cheese.

COOK'S TIP ON RED POTATOES

Be sure to use red potatoes in this recipe. They are considerably moister and hold their shape better than other varieties.

(PER SERVING)

Calories 181

Protein 13 g

Carbohydrates 25 g

Cholesterol 21 mg

Total Fat 4 g

　Saturated 2 g

　Polyunsaturated 0 g

　Monounsaturated 1 g

Fiber 4 g

Sodium 468 mg

Sweet-and-Sour Black-Eyed Peas with Ham

■ Serves 4; 1 cup per serving

■ Preparation time: 5 minutes

■ Cooking time: 5 minutes

If you've been on the lookout for new ways to use leftover ham, here's a main dish to try. Pineapple slices are a great complement as a side dish or for dessert. Substitute a flavored mustard, such as orange, horseradish, or honey mustard, for spicy brown mustard if you wish.

2 15.5-ounce cans no-salt-added black-eyed peas, rinsed and drained

1 cup low-fat, lower-sodium ham, all visible fat removed, cut into ¾-inch cubes (about 4 ounces)

3 tablespoons all-fruit black cherry spread

2 tablespoons light brown sugar

1 tablespoon plus 1½ teaspoons spicy brown mustard

1 tablespoon cider vinegar

⅛ teaspoon salt

⅛ teaspoon pepper

2 tablespoons snipped fresh parsley (optional)

In a medium saucepan, stir together all ingredients except parsley. Heat, uncovered, over medium heat for 5 minutes, or until mixture is warmed through, stirring occasionally.

Sprinkle with parsley.

(PER SERVING)

Calories 294

Protein 18 g

Carbohydrates 54 g

Cholesterol 14 mg

Total Fat 2 g

  Saturated 0 g

  Polyunsaturated —

  Monounsaturated —

Fiber 7 g

Sodium 480 mg

Ham and Hash Brown Casserole

Serves 4; 1¼ cups per serving ■
Preparation time: 15 minutes ■
Baking time: 55 minutes *or* ■
Microwave time: 16 minutes

Combine leftover ham with frozen hash browns and get an incredibly easy casserole to serve for brunch or dinner.

Vegetable oil spray

12 ounces frozen nonfat hash brown potatoes

4 ounces low-fat, lower-sodium ham, thinly sliced and chopped (about 1 cup)

1 cup frozen chopped onion, thawed, or 2 medium onions, chopped

½ cup chopped green onions (green and white parts) (about 9 green onions) or frozen or fresh green bell pepper

½ cup nonfat or light sour cream

½ cup fat-free evaporated milk or fat-free half and half

1 finely chopped jalapeño pepper or ⅛ to ¼ teaspoon cayenne (optional)

¼ teaspoon pepper

3 ounces shredded reduced-fat sharp Cheddar cheese (about ¼ cup)

Preheat oven to 350° F. Spray a 9-inch square glass baking dish with vegetable oil spray.

In a large bowl, stir together all ingredients except cheese. Pour into baking dish.

Bake for 50 minutes, or until potatoes are tender. Stir in half the cheese; sprinkle with remaining cheese. Bake for 5 minutes, or until cheese has melted.

Microwave Method

In a 9-inch microwave-safe baking dish, combine all ingredients except cheese. Cook, covered, on 100 percent power (high) for 15 minutes, or until potatoes are tender, stirring every 5 minutes. Sprinkle with cheese. Cook, uncovered, on 100 percent power (high) for 1 minute, or until cheese has melted.

(PER SERVING)

Calories 239

Protein 17 g

Carbohydrates 30 g

Cholesterol 30 mg

Total Fat 5 g

   Saturated 3 g

   Polyunsaturated 0 g

   Monounsaturated 1 g

Fiber 3 g

Sodium 471 mg

Smoked Sausage Skillet Supper

- Serves 4; 1 cup per serving
- Preparation time: 5 minutes
- Cooking time: 20 to 30 minutes

Today's nonfat and low-fat sausages make it easy to enjoy some Eastern European dishes, such as this one, that used to be hard to fit into heart-healthy eating plans.

7½ ounces precooked low-fat smoked sausage ring

Vegetable oil spray

1 tablespoon acceptable vegetable oil

½ cup frozen chopped onion or 1 medium onion, chopped

1 teaspoon bottled minced garlic or 2 medium cloves garlic, minced

3 cups fat-free frozen cubed hash brown potatoes or 4 medium potatoes, peeled and diced (about 1 pound)

14.5-ounce can no-salt-added stewed tomatoes

4 cups shredded cabbage or coleslaw mix (about 8 ounces)

⅛ to ¼ teaspoon crushed red pepper flakes

½ cup dry white wine (regular or nonalcoholic) or water

Cut sausage lengthwise into quarters, then crosswise into ¼- to ½-inch slices.

Heat a Dutch oven over medium-high heat. Remove from heat and spray with vegetable oil spray. Add oil and swirl to coat bottom of pot. Put sausage in pot; return to stovetop.

Stir in remaining ingredients except wine. Reduce heat to medium-low and cook, covered, for 10 minutes.

Stir in wine and cook for 10 minutes, or until potatoes are tender, scraping bottom of pan several times to dislodge any browned matter. Spoon extra juices over meat and vegetables.

(PER SERVING)

Calories 244

Protein 10 g

Carbohydrates 32 g

Cholesterol 24 mg

Total Fat 6 g

  Saturated 2 g

  Polyunsaturated 2 g

  Monounsaturated 1 g

Fiber 4 g

Sodium 477 mg

Curried Lamb Stew with Chick-Peas

Serves 4; 1 cup per serving ■

Preparation time: 5 minutes ■

Slow-cooker time: 4 to 5 hours on high or 8 to 9 hours on low *or* ■
Cooking time: 1 hour 36 minutes to 1 hour 38 minutes

Brinjal pickle, a zesty eggplant relish, imparts an interesting flavor into this stew. Melon slices make a nice dessert after this hearty dish.

1 pound lean boneless lamb stew meat (from leg, loin, or shoulder arm chops), all visible fat removed

Olive oil spray (stovetop method only)

½ cup frozen chopped onion or 1 medium onion, diced

1 teaspoon bottled minced garlic or 2 medium cloves garlic, minced

2 cups low-sodium chicken broth

15-ounce can no-salt-added chick-peas, rinsed and drained

2 tablespoons brinjal pickle or chutney (optional)

½ teaspoon curry powder

¼ teaspoon salt

⅛ to ¼ teaspoon crushed red pepper flakes

⅛ teaspoon black pepper

Slow-Cooker Method

Combine all ingredients (except olive oil spray) in a 3½- to 4-quart electric slow cooker. Cook, covered, on high for 4 to 5 hours or on low for 8 to 9 hours.

Stovetop Method

Heat a large, deep skillet over medium-high heat. Remove from heat and lightly spray with olive oil spray. Cook lamb cubes for 3 to 4 minutes, or until lightly browned, stirring occasionally.

Add onion and garlic; cook for 2 to 3 minutes, or until onion is tender, stirring occasionally.

Add remaining ingredients and bring to a simmer. Reduce heat to medium-low and cook, covered, for 1½ hours, or until meat is tender, stirring occasionally.

(PER SERVING)

Calories 295

Protein 28 g

Carbohydrates 22 g

Cholesterol 65 mg

Total Fat 10 g

Saturated 3 g

Polyunsaturated 1 g

Monounsaturated 3 g

Fiber 9 g

Sodium 259 mg

French Veal Stew

- Serves 6; 1⅓ cups per serving
- Preparation time: 20 minutes
- Cooking time: 27 to 30 minutes

Crumb-sprinkled veal roll-ups provide an interesting base for this unusual stew.

1 pound veal scaloppine

¼ cup plain bread crumbs

½ teaspoon salt-free Italian seasoning

Vegetable oil spray

2 teaspoons olive oil

2 cups low-sodium chicken broth

3 tablespoons all-purpose flour

1 cup baby carrots (about 8 ounces)

½ cup dry white wine (regular or nonalcoholic)

1 teaspoon dried thyme, crumbled

1 teaspoon bottled minced garlic or 2 medium cloves garlic, minced

8 ounces fresh whole mushrooms

14.5-ounce can quartered sweet potatoes, drained

1 cup frozen peas

1 cup frozen pearl onions (about 4 ounces), 14.5-ounce can pearl onions, drained, or 1 cup frozen chopped onion

¼ cup nonfat or light sour cream

Put veal in a single layer on a flat surface. Sprinkle with bread crumbs and Italian seasoning. Starting at short end, roll up jelly-roll style. Secure each roll-up with a wooden toothpick; set aside.

Heat a Dutch oven (preferably *not* nonstick) over medium-high heat. Remove from heat and spray with vegetable oil spray. Add oil and swirl to coat bottom of pot. Cook scaloppine for 4 minutes, carefully turning after each side is browned.

Meanwhile, in a medium bowl, whisk together broth and flour. When meat is browned, stir in broth mixture, carrots, wine, thyme, and garlic. Bring to a simmer over medium-high heat, 1 to 2 minutes. Reduce heat to medium-low and cook, covered, for 15 minutes (no stirring needed).

Meanwhile, trim mushrooms. Stir into pot with meat mixture as soon as they're ready.

After meat has cooked, add sweet potatoes, peas, and

onions. Cook, covered, for 5 minutes, or until vegetables and meat are tender.

Put sour cream in a small bowl. Stir in a small amount of stew; stir mixture into pan. Cook over medium-low heat for 1 to 2 minutes, or until mixture is warmed through, stirring occasionally.

FRENCH TURKEY STEW

Substitute 1 pound turkey scaloppine for veal. Serves 6; 1⅓ cups per serving. (Calories 250; Protein 23 g; Carbohydrates 29 g; Cholesterol 48 mg; Total Fat 3 g; Saturated 1 g; Polyunsaturated 1 g; Monounsaturated 1 g; Fiber 4 g; Sodium 270 mg)

(PER SERVING)

Calories 279

Protein 21 g

Carbohydrates 29 g

Cholesterol 59 mg

Total Fat 8 g

  Saturated 2 g

   Polyunsaturated 1 g

   Monounsaturated 3 g

Fiber 4 g

Sodium 287 mg

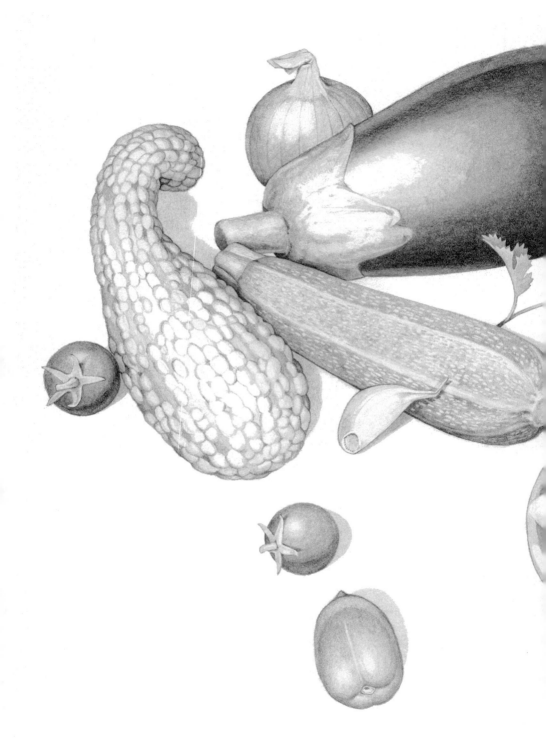

VEGETARIAN ENTRÉES

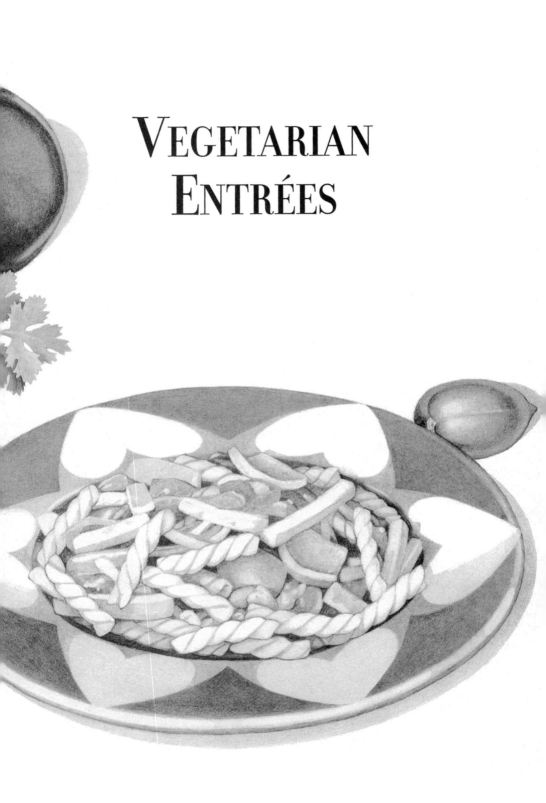

Portobello Pizza
with Peppery Greens

Provençal Pizza

Pita Pizzas

Pasta with Italian Vegetables

Italian Vegetable Stew

Italian Vegetable Stew
with Pasta

Italian Vegetables

Oven-Roasted Vegetables
and Pasta

Rosemary Peas and Pasta

Rigatoni with Cauliflower
and Tomato Sauce

Tofu Cacciatore

Exotic Mushroom Stroganoff

Mushroom-Spinach Stroganoff

Spinach Stroganoff

Pasta with Kale
and Sun-Dried Tomatoes

Vegetables in Thai Sauce
with Jasmine Rice

Brown Rice and Quinoa Pilaf

Tex-Mex Pilaf

Adzuki Beans and Rice

Black Beans and Rice

Black Bean and Rice Salad

Green Chile, Black Bean, and
Corn Stew

Bean and Vegetable Burgers

Vegetarian Chili

Greek White Beans

Red Lentils with Vegetables
and Brown Rice

Southwestern Posole Stew

Farmers' Market Stovetop
Casserole

Broccoli Potato Frittata

Spanish Tortilla

Pasta Frittata

Cajun Frittata with Pasta

Italian Gnocchi with Vegetables

Gnocchi with Italian Turkey
Sausage and Vegetables

Mozzarella Polenta with Roasted
Vegetable Salsa

Mushroom Quesadillas

Portobello Pizza with Peppery Greens

Serves 4; 1 pizza per serving ■
Preparation time: 10 minutes ■
Cooking time: 15 minutes ■

No kneading or rising time is required for this mushroom-based pizza. Place it on a bed of arugula and watercress flavored with a feta dressing, and serve as they do in Europe—with a knife and fork.

4 fresh portobello mushrooms, stems removed

Olive oil spray

Vinaigrette

2 tablespoons crumbled feta cheese, rinsed

2 tablespoons white wine vinegar

2½ teaspoons olive oil

½ to 1 teaspoon sugar

■ ■ ■

2 cups arugula leaves

2 cups watercress leaves

2 medium Italian plum tomatoes

¼ cup roasted red bell peppers, rinsed and drained

½ cup shredded mozzarella-type soy cheese or nonfat or part-skim mozzarella cheese

2 tablespoons sliced black olives

½ teaspoon dried oregano, crumbled

Preheat oven to 400° F.

Lightly spray both sides of mushrooms with olive oil spray. Place smooth side down on a nonstick baking sheet.

Bake for 10 minutes, or until mushrooms are tender.

Meanwhile, in a large bowl, whisk together vinaigrette ingredients. Add arugula and watercress; toss. Put 1 cup salad mixture on each of four plates; set aside.

Thinly slice tomatoes and peppers. Place tomato slices on baked mushrooms. Sprinkle with peppers and remaining ingredients.

Bake for 5 minutes, or until cheese is melted. Place a pizza on each salad.

(PER SERVING)

Calories 103

Protein 6 g

Carbohydrates 7 g

Cholesterol 3 mg

Total Fat 6 g

   Saturated 1 g

    Polyunsaturated 2 g

    Monounsaturated 3 g

Fiber 1 g

Sodium 292 mg

Provençal Pizza

- Serves 4; ¼ pizza per serving
- Preparation time: 5 minutes
- Cooking time: 5 minutes

Almost everyone loves pizza, but the fat grams can go through the roof. Not with this version, flavored with robust feta cheese and fresh basil. This recipe makes great use of the vegetable mixture you saved from Farmers' Market Stovetop Casserole.

16-ounce prepared pizza crust

4 medium Italian plum tomatoes, thinly sliced crosswise (13 to 14 ounces)

2 tablespoons finely chopped fresh basil or 2 teaspoons dried, crumbled

2 cups reserved vegetable mixture from Farmers' Market Stovetop Casserole (page 255)

3 ounces feta cheese, rinsed and crumbled

Preheat oven to 450° F.

Put pizza crust on baking sheet. Arrange tomato slices on crust, sprinkle basil over tomatoes, and top with vegetable mixture.

Bake for 5 minutes, or until crust is light golden brown. Sprinkle with feta.

COOK'S TIP

For a creamier texture, add feta before baking the pizza.

(PER SERVING)

Calories 400

Protein 14 g

Carbohydrates 76 g

Cholesterol 19 mg

Total Fat 5 g

  Saturated 3 g

  Polyunsaturated 0 g

  Monounsaturated 1 g

Fiber 7 g

Sodium 394 mg

Pita Pizzas

Serves 4; 1 per serving ■
Preparation time: 10 minutes ■
Cooking time: 4 to 6 minutes ■

Pita bread provides the crispy background for the perfect thin-crust pizza. For a party, add bell peppers, onions, mushrooms, broccoli, artichokes, cooked ground turkey breast, and other healthful ingredients, and let your guests create their own combinations. It's as much fun to put the pizzas together as it is to eat them.

½ cup no-salt-added tomato sauce or pizza sauce

⅛ teaspoon sugar (if using tomato sauce)

½ teaspoon dried oregano, crumbled (if using tomato sauce)

2 6-inch whole-wheat or plain pita pockets, split open into rounds

1 cup grated fat-free mozzarella-style soy cheese or part-skim mozzarella cheese (4 ounces)

½ cup thinly sliced green bell pepper

5-ounce can sliced mushrooms, rinsed and drained

1 teaspoon dried oregano, crumbled

Preheat broiler.

In a small bowl, combine tomato sauce, sugar, and ½ teaspoon oregano.

To assemble, place 2 pita halves in center of a large baking sheet. Place remaining pita halves on another baking sheet. Spread 2 tablespoons sauce on each pita, sprinkle with cheese, top with peppers and mushrooms, and sprinkle with 1 teaspoon oregano.

Place oven rack 3 to 4 inches from heat. Put one baking sheet in oven so pizzas are under flame. Broil for 2 to 3 minutes, or until cheese melts and edges begin to brown. Remove and cook remaining pizzas.

(PER SERVING)

Calories 143

Protein 11 g

Carbohydrates 23 g

Cholesterol 0 mg

Total Fat 1 g

  Saturated 0 g

  Polyunsaturated 0 g

  Monounsaturated 0 g

Fiber 3 g

Sodium 414 mg

Pasta with Italian Vegetables

- Serves 5; 1½ cups per serving
- Preparation time: 15 minutes
- Cooking time: 25 minutes

With its Old World flavors and tempting aroma, this versatile dish is a big hit at potluck suppers. Depending on whether you use the main recipe or one of the variations, you can create an entrée, a one-dish meal, or a side dish from the same basic ingredients.

8 ounces zucchini (2 small), cut into ⅛-inch slices (about 1½ cups)

8 ounces eggplant, diced (about 1½ cups)

8 ounces presliced fresh mushrooms

2 14.5-ounce cans no-salt-added diced tomatoes

1 cup frozen diced green bell pepper or 1 large green bell pepper, diced

1 tablespoon dried oregano, crumbled

1 teaspoon sugar

¼ teaspoon salt

6 ounces dried penne pasta

¼ teaspoon salt

1 tablespoon extra-virgin olive oil

In a Dutch oven, combine zucchini, eggplant, mushrooms, undrained tomatoes, bell pepper, oregano, sugar, and ¼ teaspoon salt; bring to a boil over high heat. Reduce heat and simmer, covered, for 25 minutes, or until vegetables are tender.

Meanwhile, prepare pasta using package directions, omitting salt and oil. Drain well; pour onto platter.

Remove Dutch oven from heat and stir in remaining ¼ teaspoon salt. Spoon cooked vegetable mixture over pasta and drizzle with oil.

ITALIAN VEGETABLE STEW

Omit penne pasta and olive oil. Reduce salt to ¼ teaspoon. After vegetables are cooked and salt is added, top each portion with ¼ cup shredded nonfat or part-skim mozzarella cheese (4 ounces total). Serves 4; 1½ cups per serving. (Calories 138; Protein 14 g; Carbohydrates 20 g; Cholesterol 5 mg; Total Fat 1 g; Saturated 0 g; Polyunsaturated 0 g; Monounsaturated 0 g; Fiber 6 g; Sodium 465 mg)

Italian Vegetable Stew with Pasta

Replace zucchini with a 16-ounce can no-salt-added green beans, drained. Omit olive oil. Prepare 6 ounces uncooked penne pasta as directed above; drain well and pour into a 12 x 8 x 2-inch broilerproof baking dish. Spoon cooked vegetable mixture evenly over all, and top with 6 ounces shredded part-skim or nonfat mozzarella cheese. Run under preheated broiler at least 5 inches from heat for 2 to 3 minutes, or until cheese is bubbly and beginning to lightly brown. Serves 6; 1 cup per serving. (Calories 231; Protein 12 g; Carbohydrates 38 g; Cholesterol 11 mg; Total Fat 4 g; Saturated 2 g; Polyunsaturated 1 g; Monounsaturated 1 g; Fiber 6 g; Sodium 303 mg)

Italian Vegetables

Omit penne pasta and increase olive oil to 2 tablespoons. After cooking vegetables, remove from heat and stir in oil with the ¼ teaspoon salt. Serves 12; ½ cup per serving. (Calories 52; Protein 1 g; Carbohydrates 7 g; Cholesterol 0 mg; Total Fat 3 g; Saturated 0 g; Polyunsaturated 0 g; Monounsaturated 2 g; Fiber 2 g; Sodium 107 mg)

Cook's Tip on Salt

The addition of salt near the end of preparation heightens the flavors without adding too much sodium.

(PER SERVING)

Calories 228

Protein 8 g

Carbohydrates 41 g

Cholesterol 0 mg

Total Fat 4 g

  Saturated 1 g

  Polyunsaturated 1 g

  Monounsaturated 2 g

Fiber 6 g

Sodium 258 mg

Oven-Roasted Vegetables and Pasta

- Serves 6; 1¼ cups per serving
- Preparation time: 20 minutes
- Cooking time: 15 minutes

Roasting vegetables usually takes 45 minutes or longer. This quick-roasting technique takes only 15 minutes, yet provides excellent slow-roasted flavor.

4 to 6 ounces dried rotini or other pasta

Vegetable oil spray

1 pound crookneck squash or 8 ounces crookneck squash and 8 ounces zucchini, cut into matchstick strips (3 medium)

2 medium onions, cut into eighths and then in half crosswise (yellow preferred) (½ to ¾ pound)

1 medium green bell pepper, cut into 1-inch squares

8 ounces cherry tomatoes, halved

¼ cup finely chopped fresh basil or 1 tablespoon plus 1½ teaspoons dried, crumbled

1½ tablespoons cider vinegar or balsamic vinegar

1 tablespoon extra-virgin olive oil

2 teaspoons bottled minced garlic or 4 medium cloves garlic, minced

3 ounces feta cheese, rinsed and crumbled

½ teaspoon salt

⅛ to ¼ teaspoon crushed red pepper flakes

Cook pasta using package directions, omitting salt and oil.

Meanwhile, preheat broiler. Line a large broiler pan or two baking sheets with aluminum foil. Spray foil with vegetable oil spray. Put squash, onions, peppers, and tomatoes in broiler pan.

Broil about 5 inches from heat for 15 minutes, or until edges are brown and peppers are just tender, stirring every 5 minutes.

Meanwhile, in a small bowl, whisk together basil, vinegar, oil, and garlic.

Drain pasta and put in a large bowl. Gently stir in all ingredients.

COOK'S TIP

Omit the pasta and serve this as a side dish.

(PER SERVING)

Calories 189

Protein 7 g

Carbohydrates 28 g

Cholesterol 13 mg

Total Fat 6 g

  Saturated 3 g

  Polyunsaturated 1 g

  Monounsaturated 2 g

Fiber 3 g

Sodium 360 mg

Rosemary Peas and Pasta

Serves 8; 1½ cups per serving ■
Preparation time: 5 minutes ■
Cooking time: 15 minutes ■

Keep these ingredients on hand so you can have a tempting, inexpensive entrée ready in almost no time.

12 ounces dried medium pasta shells

1 tablespoon extra-virgin olive oil

20-ounce bag frozen green peas (4 cups)

¾ cup frozen chopped onion or 1 large onion, coarsely chopped (sweet preferred)

2 tablespoons bottled minced garlic or 12 medium cloves garlic, minced

1 teaspoon dried rosemary, crushed

¼ teaspoon crushed red pepper flakes

½ teaspoon black pepper

3 tablespoons shredded or grated Parmesan cheese

Cook pasta using package directions, omitting salt and oil. Reserve 2 cups cooking liquid; drain pasta and leave in colander.

Meanwhile, heat a large skillet over medium heat. Add oil and swirl to coat bottom of skillet. Cook peas, onion, garlic, rosemary, and red pepper flakes, covered, for 7 to 10 minutes, stirring occasionally.

Stir in reserved cooking liquid and black pepper. Cook, covered, for 3 minutes, stirring occasionally.

To serve, transfer pasta to a large serving bowl; stir in pea mixture. Sprinkle with Parmesan.

(PER SERVING)

Calories 251

Protein 10 g

Carbohydrates 44 g

Cholesterol 2 mg

Total Fat 4 g

 Saturated 1 g

 Polyunsaturated 1 g

 Monounsaturated 2 g

Fiber 5 g

Sodium 123 mg

Rigatoni with Cauliflower and Tomato Sauce

- Serves 8; 2 cups per serving
- Preparation time: 10 minutes
- Cooking time: 29 to 34 minutes

To vary this flavorful dish, serve the sauce over another kind of pasta or brown rice. It's even delicious over toasted Italian bread, or if you have leftovers, add crumbled fat-free veggie burgers or part-skim or nonfat mozzarella cheese.

1 pound dried rigatoni

Cauliflower and Tomato Sauce

2 tablespoons extra-virgin olive oil

20-ounce bag frozen no-salt-added cauliflower florets (4 cups)

1 large sweet onion, coarsely chopped (about ¾ cup)

1 cup coarsely snipped fresh parsley (Italian, or flat-leaf, preferred)

¼ cup coarsely chopped fresh basil

2 to 3 tablespoons bottled minced garlic or 12 to 18 medium cloves garlic, finely chopped

¼ cup dry red wine (regular or nonalcoholic)

2 cups water

32 ounces marinara sauce

⅛ teaspoon cayenne

Freshly ground black pepper

■ ■ ■

3 tablespoons shredded or grated Parmesan cheese

(PER SERVING)

Calories 357

Protein 13 g

Carbohydrates 57 g

Cholesterol 2 mg

Total Fat 8 g

Saturated 1 g

Polyunsaturated —

Monounsaturated —

Fiber 5 g

Sodium 281 mg

Cook pasta using package directions, omitting salt and oil; drain and set aside.

Meanwhile, heat a 4- to 6-quart pot or a Dutch oven over medium heat. Add oil and swirl to coat bottom of pot. Cook cauliflower, onion, parsley, basil, and garlic, covered, for 10 minutes, or until vegetables release some of their liquids, stirring occasionally.

Stir in remaining sauce ingredients. Cover and increase heat to medium-high; bring to a boil. Cook, covered, at a medium boil for 12 to 15 minutes, or until cauliflower is tender, stirring occasionally.

Turn cooked pasta into a large serving bowl. Spoon half the sauce over pasta; using two spoons, toss to coat. Spoon remaining sauce over pasta. Sprinkle with Parmesan.

Tofu Cacciatore

Serves 5; 1½ cups per serving ■
Preparation time: 15 minutes ■
Cooking time: 25 to 30 minutes ■

For a delicious Italian dinner, serve this flavorful combination of mushrooms, peppers, and tomatoes with brown rice or on your favorite pasta.

1 tablespoon plus 1 teaspoon extra-virgin olive oil

2 large bell peppers, cut into ½-inch strips (red, yellow, or green)

4 to 6 ounces presliced fresh portobello mushrooms

1 large onion (sweet preferred), cut vertically into thick slices, or ¾ cup frozen chopped onion

1 large carrot, finely chopped

2 teaspoons bottled minced garlic or 4 medium cloves garlic, minced

28-ounce can no-salt-added whole peeled Italian plum tomatoes

¼ cup dry red wine (regular or nonalcoholic)

1 teaspoon dried oregano, crumbled

1 teaspoon dried thyme, crumbled

¼ teaspoon pepper

12- to 14-ounce package low-fat extra-firm tofu

Heat a 12-inch skillet or Dutch oven over medium-high heat. Add oil. Stir in bell peppers, mushrooms, onion, carrot, and garlic, coating with oil. Cook, covered, for 5 to 7 minutes, or until peppers soften and release some of their juices, stirring occasionally.

Stir in remaining ingredients except tofu. Using a spoon, cut tomatoes into large pieces. Cover skillet, increase heat to high, and bring to a medium-high boil. Reduce heat to medium-high and cook for 10 to 12 minutes, or until peppers are soft, stirring occasionally.

Meanwhile, drain tofu if necessary. Cut into small cubes. Stir into vegetable mixture and cook for 5 minutes, or until hot, stirring occasionally.

(PER SERVING)

Calories 152

Protein 8 g

Carbohydrates 17 g

Cholesterol 0 mg

Total Fat 5 g

   Saturated 1 g

   Polyunsaturated 1 g

   Monounsaturated 3 g

Fiber 4 g

Sodium 81 mg

Exotic Mushroom Stroganoff

- Serves 4; 1½ cups per serving
- Preparation time: 20 minutes
- Cooking time: 20 minutes

No one will ask "Where's the beef?" when eating this stroganoff. The sauce is rich with a variety of mushrooms, as well as marsala and dill. For a change, try it with rice or Bean and Vegetable Burgers (page 250), or even store-bought veggie burgers.

8 ounces dried pasta, such as yolk-free noodles

1 tablespoon olive oil

¾ cup frozen chopped onion or 1 large onion, thinly sliced

4- to 6-ounce package presliced fresh portobello mushrooms

1 to 1¼ pounds mixed fresh mushrooms, such as cremini, portobello, and shiitake, cut into ¼-inch slices

2 teaspoons dried dillweed, crumbled

1 teaspoon bottled minced garlic or 2 medium cloves garlic, minced

⅛ to ¼ teaspoon pepper

8 ounces nonfat sour cream (1 cup)

8 ounces light sour cream (1 cup)

¼ cup dry marsala or dry sherry

¾ teaspoon paprika

Prepare pasta using package directions, omitting salt and oil; drain well.

Meanwhile, heat a large skillet over low-medium heat. Add oil and swirl to coat bottom of skillet. Cook onions, mushrooms, dillweed, garlic, and pepper, covered, for 15 minutes, stirring occasionally.

In a small bowl, whisk together remaining ingredients. Whisk in several spoonfuls of hot mushroom mixture. Stir sour cream mixture into skillet; cook for 3 minutes, or until heated through. Don't let mixture come to a boil, or sour cream will curdle.

To serve, transfer pasta to a serving dish. Spoon sauce over pasta.

MUSHROOM-SPINACH STROGANOFF

Replace half the mushrooms with 10 ounces fresh spinach. (Calories 411; Protein 19 g; Carbohydrates 66 g; Cholesterol 24 mg; Total Fat 8 g; Saturated 3 g;

Polyunsaturated 1 g; Monounsaturated 4 g; Fiber 4 g; Sodium 208 mg)

SPINACH STROGANOFF

Replace all the mushrooms with 1¼ pounds fresh spinach. (Calories 407; Protein 19 g; Carbohydrates 66 g; Cholesterol 24 mg; Total Fat 9 g; Saturated 3 g; Polyunsaturated 1 g; Monounsaturated 4 g; Fiber 6 g; Sodium 264 mg)

COOK'S TIP

If you can't find several varieties of exotic mushroom, you can substitute button mushrooms. The finished dish won't be quite as rich, but it will still be delicious.

(PER SERVING)

Calories 419
Protein 18 g
Carbohydrates 69 g
Cholesterol 24 mg
Total Fat 8 g
  Saturated 3 g
  Polyunsaturated 1 g
  Monounsaturated 4 g
Fiber 3 g
Sodium 154 mg

Pasta with Kale and Sun-Dried Tomatoes

- Serves 5; 1½ cups per serving
- Preparation time: 20 minutes
- Cooking time: 22 minutes

Serve this as a vegetarian entrée or as a side dish with baked chicken. The cheese or olives lend a little pungent punch and counteract the sweetness of the dried tomatoes.

1 ounce sun-dried tomatoes, dry-packed (⅓ cup)

½ cup boiling water

1 bunch kale (about 10 ounces)

16 ounces dried medium pasta shells

2 teaspoons olive oil

2 teaspoons minced garlic or 4 medium cloves garlic, minced

¼ teaspoon crushed red pepper flakes

3 ounces crumbled feta, rinsed, or blue cheese or ¼ cup minced green olives or imported black olives, such as kalamata or niçoise

Put tomatoes in a small bowl and pour in boiling water; set aside.

Remove thick stems from kale. Roughly cut leaves into about ¼-inch strips; set aside.

Cook pasta using package directions, omitting salt and oil, until still firm when you bite into it (start tasting 3 minutes before package says it will be done); drain.

Meanwhile, heat a large skillet over medium heat. Add oil and swirl to coat bottom of skillet. Cook garlic and red pepper until garlic becomes aromatic and begins to brown, 30 to 60 seconds.

Stir kale into skillet.

Drain tomatoes, combining soaking liquid with enough water to equal ¾ cup. Pour into skillet. Chop tomatoes and stir into kale mixture; bring to a boil. Reduce heat and simmer, covered, for 5 to 10 minutes, or until greens have wilted and are slightly tender.

To serve, combine pasta and kale mixture. Spoon onto plates or platter and sprinkle with cheese.

COOK'S TIP ON KALE

Some supermarkets carry prewashed kale. If you find it, you can cut your prep time by about 15 minutes.

(PER SERVING)

Calories 429

Protein 17 g

Carbohydrates 78 g

Cholesterol 15 mg

Total Fat 7 g

Saturated 3 g

Polyunsaturated 0 g

Monounsaturated 2 g

Fiber 4 g

Sodium 340 mg

VEGETARIAN ENTRÉES

Vegetables in Thai Sauce with Jasmine Rice

Serves 5; 1 cup vegetables and ½ cup rice per serving ■
Preparation time: 5 minutes ■
Cooking time: 28 to 38 minutes ■

❶

This Thai dish has the traditional flavor combination of basil, peanut, and coconut made with the convenience of a store-bought peanut satay sauce. Jasmine rice has a light floral aroma and is a welcome change from everyday rice.

1 cup uncooked jasmine rice

1 teaspoon acceptable vegetable oil

2 16-ounce packages frozen mixed stir-fry vegetables

½ cup coarsely chopped fresh basil

2 tablespoons bottled minced garlic or 12 medium cloves garlic, minced

¼ teaspoon crushed red pepper flakes

2 cups fat-free milk

7-ounce jar peanut satay sauce

2 tablespoons lime juice (1 to 2 medium limes)

Prepare rice using package directions, omitting salt and margarine.

Meanwhile, heat oil in a large saucepan over medium heat. Stir in vegetables, basil, garlic, and red pepper flakes. Cook, covered, for 12 to 15 minutes, or until vegetables are heated through, stirring occasionally.

Stir in milk, satay sauce, and lime juice. Cook, covered, for 3 to 5 minutes, or until heated through, stirring occasionally.

Serve over rice.

(PER SERVING)

Calories 313

Protein 8 g

Carbohydrates 56 g

Cholesterol 2 mg

Total Fat 7 g

  Saturated 0 g

  Polyunsaturated —

  Monounsaturated —

Fiber 6 g

Sodium 173 mg

Brown Rice and Quinoa Pilaf

- Serves 5; 1 cup per serving
- Preparation time: 5 minutes
- Cooking time: 17 to 20 minutes

Nutrient-packed, quinoa contains complete protein, making it a wise choice for quick cooks. Steam some asparagus and slice some fruit, and dinner is ready.

¼ cup quinoa, rinsed and drained

1 tablespoon sliced almonds

Olive oil spray

1 cup presliced fresh mushrooms (3 ounces)

½ cup shredded carrots

2 cups uncooked instant brown rice

½ cup carrot juice

1¾ cups water

1 teaspoon onion powder

½ teaspoon dried thyme, crumbled

¼ teaspoon salt

⅛ teaspoon pepper

1 cup frozen peas

1 teaspoon lemon zest (optional)

Preheat a medium nonstick saucepan over medium-high heat. Cook quinoa and almonds for 3 to 4 minutes, or until lightly toasted, stirring occasionally. Pour mixture into a small bowl and set aside.

Lightly spray same saucepan with olive oil spray. Put saucepan back over medium-high heat. Cook mushrooms and carrots for 2 to 3 minutes, or until tender.

Stir in quinoa mixture, rice, carrot juice, water, onion powder, thyme, salt, and pepper; bring to a boil over high heat. Reduce heat to low and cook, covered, for 10 minutes.

Stir in peas and lemon zest; cook for 3 to 4 minutes, or until quinoa and rice are tender. Serve warm.

(PER SERVING)

Calories 230

Protein 7 g

Carbohydrates 47 g

Cholesterol 0 mg

Total Fat 3 g

  Saturated 0 g

  Polyunsaturated 1 g

  Monounsaturated 1 g

Fiber 4 g

Sodium 179 mg

Tex-Mex Pilaf

Serves 4; 1¼ cups per serving ■
Preparation time: 5 minutes ■
Cooking time: 40 minutes ■

One-pot meals, such as this vegetarian pilaf, are fabulous time-savers and require little energy. If you wish, add a little chopped skinless chicken or lean, low-sodium ham with the other ingredients.

2 teaspoons olive oil

½ cup frozen chopped onion or
   1 medium onion, chopped

15-ounce can no-salt-added kidney
   beans, rinsed and drained

1¼ cups water or low-sodium chicken
   broth

1 cup uncooked rice

1 cup fresh or frozen no-salt-added
   whole-kernel corn

1 cup chunky salsa

¼ cup lentils, sorted for stones and
   shriveled lentils and rinsed

¼ cup chopped red bell pepper or
   canned pimiento, drained

½ teaspoon chili powder, or to taste

¼ teaspoon crushed red pepper flakes,
   or to taste

Dash garlic powder (optional)

Heat a heavy 2-quart saucepan over medium-high heat. Add oil and swirl to coat bottom of pan. Cook onion for 2 minutes, or until translucent, stirring occasionally.

Stir in remaining ingredients; bring to a boil over high heat. Reduce heat to low and cook, covered, for 30 minutes, or until lentils and rice are cooked through.

(PER SERVING)

Calories 375

Protein 14 g

Carbohydrates 72 g

Cholesterol 0 mg

Total Fat 4 g

  Saturated 1 g

   Polyunsaturated 1 g

   Monounsaturated 2 g

Fiber 11 g

Sodium 359 mg

Adzuki Beans and Rice

- Serves 4; ¼ cup rice and ⅓ cup beans per serving
- Preparation time: 10 minutes
- Cooking time: 17 to 19 minutes

❶

Asian adzuki beans and fresh mushrooms contrast nicely with aromatic vegetables, thyme, and cumin in this updated version of a classic dish.

Rice

1 cup fresh mushrooms (shiitake preferred)

1 teaspoon olive oil

1 rib celery, diced (about ½ cup)

⅓ cup frozen chopped onion or ⅔ medium onion, diced

¼ cup frozen chopped green bell pepper or ½ large green bell pepper, diced

1 teaspoon bottled minced garlic or 2 medium cloves garlic, minced

1½ cups instant brown rice

1¼ cups low-sodium vegetable broth

1 teaspoon dried thyme, crumbled

⅛ teaspoon crushed red pepper flakes or cayenne

Beans

15-ounce can no-salt-added adzuki beans or kidney beans, rinsed and drained

½ teaspoon ground cumin

¼ teaspoon salt

2 tablespoons snipped fresh parsley or cilantro (optional)

For rice, remove stems from mushrooms; discard stems and slice caps.

Heat a medium saucepan over medium-high heat. Add olive oil and swirl to coat bottom of pan. Cook celery, onions, bell pepper, and garlic for 2 to 3 minutes, or until tender, stirring occasionally.

Add mushrooms and cook for 1 to 2 minutes, stirring occasionally.

Stir in remaining seasoned rice ingredients; bring to a boil over high heat. Reduce heat and simmer, covered, for 5 minutes. Fluff with a fork, remove from heat, and let stand, covered, for 5 minutes.

Meanwhile, in a small saucepan, stir together beans, cumin, and salt. Cook over medium-low heat until warmed through, 3 to 4 minutes, stirring occasionally. Keep warm over low heat. (You can also put bean mix-

ture in a microwave-safe bowl, cover with vented plastic wrap, and cook on 100 percent power [high] for 2 to 3 minutes, or until warmed through.)

To serve, spoon about ¾ cup rice mixture into each bowl. Add about ⅓ cup beans and sprinkle with a small amount of parsley.

COOK'S TIP ON ADZUKI BEANS

Red bean paste, a popular ingredient in Chinese and Japanese cooking, is made from lightly sweetened adzuki beans (also spelled "aduki" and "azuki"). Whole adzuki beans have a delicate texture, mild flavor, and deep red color. You can find them in health food stores or Asian grocery stores. Use them in soups, salads, and casseroles.

(PER SERVING)
Calories 270
Protein 10 g
Carbohydrates 55 g
Cholesterol 0 mg
Total Fat 3 g
  Saturated 0 g
  Polyunsaturated 0 g
  Monounsaturated 1 g
Fiber 2 g
Sodium 185 mg

Black Beans and Rice

- Serves 6; 1 cup per serving
- Preparation time: 5 minutes
- Cooking time: 5 minutes

To jazz up black beans and rice, add the exciting flavors of rich olive oil, tangy lime juice, and assertive fresh garlic.

2 cups uncooked instant rice

2 tablespoons plus 2 teaspoons extra-virgin olive oil

¼ cup lime juice (2 to 3 medium limes)

2 medium cloves garlic, minced, or 1 teaspoon bottled minced garlic

½ teaspoon salt

15-ounce can no-salt-added black beans, rinsed and drained

2 tablespoons finely snipped fresh cilantro (optional)

Cook rice using package directions, omitting salt and margarine.

Meanwhile, in a small bowl, whisk together oil, lime juice, garlic, and salt.

Stir beans into cooked rice; transfer to serving platter. Drizzle with oil mixture, add cilantro, and stir gently.

BLACK BEAN AND RICE SALAD

For a delicious salad, cook rice as directed above; cool for 5 to 8 minutes in a thin layer on a baking sheet, stirring occasionally. Follow directions above, adding 1 cup chopped red or green bell pepper, 2 additional tablespoons lime juice, and ⅛ additional teaspoon salt. Serves 7; 1 cup per serving. (Calories 212; Protein 6 g; Carbohydrates 35 g; Cholesterol 0 mg; Total Fat 6 g; Saturated 1 g; Polyunsaturated 1 g; Monounsaturated 4 g; Fiber 3 g; Sodium 213 mg)

(PER SERVING)

Calories 241

Protein 7 g

Carbohydrates 39 g

Cholesterol 0 mg

Total Fat 6 g

Saturated 1 g

Polyunsaturated 1 g

Monounsaturated 4 g

Fiber 3 g

Sodium 198 mg

VEGETARIAN ENTRÉES

Green Chile, Black Bean, and Corn Stew

Serves 4; 1¼ cups per serving ■

Preparation time: 5 minutes ■

Cooking time: 28 minutes ■

Standing time: 5 to 10 minutes ■

If your party grows, you can stretch this hearty Southwestern stew by serving it over rice. Put about a half cup of cooked rice in each bowl, then top with the stew.

1 teaspoon extra-virgin olive oil

6 to 8 ounces Anaheim peppers, poblano peppers, or green bell pepper (1 large), chopped

2 cups frozen or canned no-salt-added whole-kernel corn, rinsed and drained if canned

15-ounce can no-salt-added black beans, rinsed and drained

14.5-ounce can no-salt-added diced tomatoes or stewed tomatoes

1 cup water

1 tablespoon chili powder

1 teaspoon ground cumin

½ teaspoon salt

Heat a Dutch oven over medium-high heat. Add oil and swirl to coat bottom of pot. Cook peppers for 6 minutes, or until tender-crisp, stirring frequently.

Stir in remaining ingredients except salt; bring to a boil. Reduce heat and simmer, covered, for 20 minutes. Remove from heat.

Stir in salt and let stand, uncovered, for 5 to 10 minutes to allow flavors to blend and stew to thicken slightly.

(PER SERVING)

Calories 224

Protein 11 g

Carbohydrates 44 g

Cholesterol 0 mg

Total Fat 3 g

  Saturated 0 g

  Polyunsaturated 1 g

  Monounsaturated 1 g

Fiber 9 g

Sodium 329 mg

Bean and Vegetable Burgers

- Serves 6; 1 burger and ½ pita bread per serving
- Preparation time: 20 minutes
- Cooking time: 6 to 8 minutes

You may want to prepare a double batch of these burgers to serve without the pita bread at another meal. Try them with roasted sweet potato wedges and fresh fruit.

Burgers

15-ounce can no-salt-added kidney beans, rinsed and drained

15-ounce can no-salt-added black beans, rinsed and drained

½ cup shredded carrots

4 green onions, thinly sliced (about ½ cup)

¼ cup plain dry bread crumbs

1 teaspoon chili powder

1 teaspoon garlic powder

¼ teaspoon salt

■ ■ ■

1 tablespoon olive oil

Olive oil spray (optional)

3 whole-wheat pita breads

6 leaves of lettuce, any variety

¾ cup salsa

In a food processor or blender, pulse kidney beans and black beans on and off for 20 to 30 seconds, until mixture is slightly chunky.

In a medium bowl, combine beans with remaining burger ingredients. Shape into six flat patties.

Heat a large skillet over medium-high heat. Add oil and swirl to coat bottom of skillet. Cook patties for 3 to 4 minutes, or until browned. Remove skillet from heat and spray tops with olive oil spray; turn patties over. Cook for 3 to 4 minutes, or until browned.

To serve, cut each pita bread in half crosswise, making two pockets. Open pita bread halves and place burgers and lettuce inside. Serve with salsa.

(PER SERVING)

Calories 274

Protein 13 g

Carbohydrates 48 g

Cholesterol 0 mg

Total Fat 4 g

  Saturated 1 g

  Polyunsaturated 1 g

  Monounsaturated 2 g

Fiber 10 g

Sodium 418 mg

Vegetarian Chili

Serves 4; 1½ cups per serving ■
Preparation time: 10 minutes ■
Cooking time: 23 to 33 minutes ■

When your meat-loving guests taste this chili, they'll be amazed that you created such a wonderful meatless dish.

1 cup no-salt-added tomato juice

½ cup bulgur

Vegetable oil spray

2 tablespoons olive oil

½ cup frozen chopped onion or
1 medium onion, chopped

2 teaspoons bottled minced garlic or
4 medium cloves garlic, minced

2 16-ounce cans no-salt-added pinto
or kidney beans

14.5-ounce can no-salt-added
crushed tomatoes

4-ounce can chopped green chiles,
rinsed and drained

2 tablespoons chili powder

1 teaspoon ground cumin

1 teaspoon dried oregano, crumbled

¼ teaspoon cayenne

1 cup water

In a medium bowl or pan, bring tomato juice to a boil in microwave or on stovetop. Add bulgur, stir several times, and set aside.

Heat a Dutch oven over medium-high heat. Remove from heat and spray with vegetable oil spray. Add olive oil and swirl to coat bottom of pot. Cook onion and garlic for about 3 minutes, or until onion is soft and garlic is aromatic, stirring occasionally.

Add remaining ingredients except water and bring to a boil over high heat.

Stir in water and bulgur mixture; return to a boil. Reduce heat and simmer, uncovered, for 10 to 20 minutes (more simmering allows the flavors to blend).

COOK'S TIP ON BULGUR

Bulgur is made of wheat berries that have been cooked and drained. It makes a good substitute for ground beef in many recipes. Bulgur soaks up liquid, so add more water for soupier chili or when reheating leftovers.

(PER SERVING)

Calories 382

Protein 14 g

Carbohydrates 63 g

Cholesterol 0 mg

Total Fat 8 g

  Saturated 1 g

   Polyunsaturated 1 g

   Monounsaturated 5 g

Fiber 17 g

Sodium 411 mg

Greek White Beans

- Serves 6; 1 cup per serving
- Preparation time: 10 minutes
- Cooking time: 16 to 21 minutes

Greeks often serve white beans on fast days as a filling and hearty alternative to meat. Good alone or served over orzo or rice, these beans have even more flavor the second day.

2 tablespoons extra-virgin olive oil

1 rib celery, chopped (about ½ cup)

1 medium carrot, chopped

½ cup frozen chopped onion or 1 medium onion, chopped

2 16-ounce cans no-salt-added navy or Great Northern beans

½ cup snipped fresh parsley

2 tablespoons no-salt-added tomato paste

1 tablespoon fresh oregano or 1 teaspoon dried, crumbled

½ teaspoon crushed red pepper flakes

½ teaspoon salt

1 teaspoon freshly ground black pepper

Heat a large saucepan over high heat. Add oil and swirl to coat bottom of pan. Cook celery, carrot, and onion until softened, 8 to 10 minutes, stirring frequently.

Add remaining ingredients; bring to a boil. Reduce heat and simmer for 5 to 8 minutes, or until heated through.

COOK'S TIP ON TOMATO PASTE

In Mediterranean cuisine, tomato paste is used sparingly. Cooks would rarely put 6 ounces in a family dish, yet most tomato paste sold in the United States comes in 6-ounce cans. If you use it all, the dish is too sweet. Instead, use a small amount for flavor, then freeze the rest. Measure 1-tablespoon portions, freeze on a baking sheet, then remove the cubes and store them in an airtight plastic bag in the freezer. The paste thaws quickly and can even be used still frozen when you're cooking.

(PER SERVING)

Calories 186

Protein 9 g

Carbohydrates 27 g

Cholesterol 0 mg

Total Fat 5 g

  Saturated 1 g

  Polyunsaturated 0 g

  Monounsaturated 3 g

Fiber 9 g

Sodium 231 mg

Red Lentils with Vegetables and Brown Rice

Serves 6; 1½ cups per serving ■
Preparation time: 5 minutes ■
Cooking time: 38 to 40 minutes ■

This dish tastes even better the second day. If you have leftovers, warm them and serve in pita pockets.

1 tablespoon olive oil

2 medium carrots, chopped

1 teaspoon bottled minced garlic or 2 medium cloves garlic, minced

5 cups water

2 cups low-sodium vegetable broth

15-ounce can no-salt-added stewed tomatoes

1 cup red lentils, sorted for stones or shriveled lentils and rinsed

1 teaspoon fennel seeds, dried basil or thyme, crumbled, or dried rosemary, crushed

1 teaspoon dried oregano, crumbled

½ teaspoon salt

⅛ teaspoon pepper

2 cups uncooked instant brown rice

Heat a large stockpot over medium-high heat. Add oil and swirl to coat bottom of pot. Cook carrots and garlic for 2 to 3 minutes, or until carrots are slightly tender.

Stir in remaining ingredients except brown rice; bring to a boil over high heat. Reduce heat to medium-low and cook, covered, for 30 minutes, or until lentils are tender.

Stir in brown rice and cook, covered, for 5 minutes, or until rice is tender.

COOK'S TIP ON RED LENTILS

Red lentils are colorful, versatile, and take less time to cook than other lentils. For an Indian-inspired dish, add 1 tablespoon fat-free salad dressing, such as Italian or balsamic vinaigrette, and ½ cup chopped raw vegetables to every ½ cup cooked and chilled red lentils.

(PER SERVING)

Calories 291

Protein 13 g

Carbohydrates 55 g

Cholesterol 0 mg

Total Fat 4 g

Saturated 1 g

Polyunsaturated —

Monounsaturated —

Fiber 13 g

Sodium 241 mg

Southwestern Posole Stew

- Serves 4; 1¼ cups per serving
- Preparation time: 5 minutes
- Cooking time: 7 to 8 minutes

 ❶

Golden hominy, which has the aroma and flavor of corn tortillas, is one of the high-lights of this zesty stew.

1 tablespoon olive oil

2 ribs celery, chopped (about 1 cup)

½ cup frozen chopped onion or
1 medium onion, chopped

1 teaspoon bottled minced garlic or
2 medium cloves garlic, minced

15-ounce can no-salt-added pinto
beans

15-ounce can golden hominy, rinsed
and drained

1 cup water

8-ounce can no-salt-added tomato
sauce (1 cup)

2 teaspoons chili powder

1 teaspoon ground cumin

⅛ teaspoon pepper

Heat a large saucepan over medium-high heat. Add oil and swirl to coat bottom of pan. Cook celery, onions, and garlic for 2 to 3 minutes, or until tender.

Add remaining ingredients and bring to a boil over high heat. Reduce heat to medium and simmer for 5 minutes, or until flavors are blended and mixture is warmed through. Ladle into bowls.

COOK'S TIP ON HOMINY

Look for canned hominy, yellow or white, near the canned corn in the supermarket.

(PER SERVING)

Calories 224

Protein 7 g

Carbohydrates 38 g

Cholesterol 0 mg

Total Fat 5 g

  Saturated 1 g

  Polyunsaturated 1 g

  Monounsaturated 3 g

Fiber 10 g

Sodium 280 mg

Farmers' Market Stovetop Casserole

Serves 4; 1¼ cups per serving (plus 2 cups reserved) ■

Preparation time: 15 minutes ■

Cooking time: 10 minutes ■

Standing time: 5 minutes ■

If you love shopping for vegetables but don't know what to do with them once you're home, this is the perfect recipe for you. You'll even have a headstart on dinner for later in the week because you save two cups of the vegetables for Provençal Pizza.

2 cups water

1 pound red potatoes, cut into 1-inch pieces

3 cups small broccoli florets (about 12 ounces)

8 ounces presliced fresh mushrooms

1 large red or green bell pepper, cut into thin strips (about 8 ounces)

2 4-ounce onions, cut into eighths (yellow preferred)

¼ cup water

⅓ cup snipped fresh parsley

½ teaspoon salt

¼ teaspoon dried thyme, crumbled

Pepper to taste

¾ cup shredded reduced-fat sharp Cheddar cheese (about 3 ounces)

Pour 2 cups water into a large saucepan. Put steam basket in pan. Put potatoes in basket; cover. Bring water to a boil over high heat. Reduce heat to a simmer and steam potatoes for 5 minutes, or until just tender.

Meanwhile, heat a Dutch oven over high heat. Put broccoli, mushrooms, bell pepper, onions, and ¼ cup water into pot; bring to a boil. Reduce heat to medium and cook, covered, for 8 to 10 minutes, or until broccoli is tender-crisp, stirring occasionally. Remove from heat. With a slotted spoon, remove 2 cups of the mixture and reserve for Provençal Pizza (page 232).

Stir potatoes, parsley, salt, thyme, and pepper into Dutch oven. Sprinkle with cheese, cover, and let stand for 5 minutes to blend flavors and melt cheese.

(PER SERVING)

Calories 191

Protein 11 g

Carbohydrates 29 g

Cholesterol 14 mg

Total Fat 4 g

Saturated 2 g

Polyunsaturated 0 g

Monounsaturated 1 g

Fiber 4 g

Sodium 447 mg

Broccoli Potato Frittata

- Serves 4; 1 wedge per serving
- Preparation time: 10 minutes
- Cooking time: 15 to 17 minutes

Choose fresh fruit salad or cold soup, such as Chilled Strawberry Orange Soup (page 63), to complement this quichelike dish.

3 cups fat-free frozen shredded hash browns

1 teaspoon olive oil

¼ cup frozen chopped onion or ½ medium onion, chopped

1 teaspoon bottled minced garlic or 2 medium cloves garlic, minced

2 cups broccoli florets, cut into ¾-inch pieces (about 8 ounces)

⅛ teaspoon pepper

Egg substitute equivalent to 4 eggs

¼ cup reduced-fat grated Cheddar cheese (about 1 ounce)

1 tablespoon plus 1½ teaspoons shredded or grated Parmesan cheese

2 medium Italian plum tomatoes, sliced (optional)

Put potatoes in a colander and rinse with warm water for 1 to 2 minutes to partially thaw. Set aside to drain.

Heat a large nonstick skillet over medium-high heat. Add oil and swirl to coat bottom of skillet. Cook onion and garlic for 2 minutes, stirring occasionally.

Add broccoli and cook for 1 minute, stirring occasionally.

Stir in potatoes, mixing well; sprinkle with pepper.

Pour egg substitute over all; sprinkle with cheeses. Reduce heat to medium-low and cook, covered, for 10 to 12 minutes, or until eggs are set.

To serve, cut into wedges and garnish with tomato slices.

(PER SERVING)

Calories 166

Protein 13 g

Carbohydrates 19 g

Cholesterol 11 mg

Total Fat 3 g

  Saturated 1 g

  Polyunsaturated 0 g

  Monounsaturated 1 g

Fiber 3 g

Sodium 227 mg

Spanish Tortilla

Serves 4; 1 wedge per serving ■
Preparation time: 5 minutes ■
Cooking time: 22 to 31 minutes ■

The tortilla is Spain's answer to Italy's frittata. By any name, this type of dish makes a fine brunch, lunch, or dinner entrée.

1 tablespoon extra-virgin olive oil

2 large potatoes, peeled and finely chopped (Yukon Gold preferred) (about 1 pound)

½ cup frozen chopped onion or 1 medium onion (sweet preferred), finely chopped

1 to 2 teaspoons water (as needed)

Egg substitute equivalent to 8 eggs

¼ teaspoon pepper

1 cup salsa

Heat olive oil in a large nonstick skillet over medium heat. Add potatoes and onion, stirring to coat. Cook, covered, for 7 to 10 minutes, or until potatoes are just tender, stirring frequently. If potatoes begin to stick or burn, add water.

Pour egg substitute evenly over potato mixture. Sprinkle with pepper. Reduce heat to medium-low and cook, covered, for 10 to 15 minutes, or until eggs are set.

Meanwhile, in a small saucepan over medium-low heat, heat salsa for 5 to 7 minutes.

Cut tortilla into four wedges and serve with heated salsa on the side.

(PER SERVING)

Calories 175

Protein 13 g

Carbohydrates 19 g

Cholesterol 0 mg

Total Fat 5 g

Saturated 1 g

Polyunsaturated 0 g

Monounsaturated 3 g

Fiber 2 g

Sodium 404 mg

Pasta Frittata

- Serves 6; 1 wedge per serving
- Preparation time: 15 minutes
- Cooking time: 16 minutes
- Standing time: 5 minutes

This mildly seasoned frittata—basically an omelet without the work—is a different way to use leftover pasta.

Vegetable oil spray

8 ounces presliced fresh mushrooms

1 cup zucchini, thinly sliced (1 medium)

1 cup frozen chopped onion or 2 medium onions, chopped (yellow preferred)

Egg substitute equivalent to 4 eggs

¼ cup fat-free milk

2 tablespoons finely snipped fresh parsley

1½ teaspoons dried oregano, crumbled

¼ teaspoon salt

2 cups cooked spaghetti or yolk-free noodles (4 ounces dried)

3 ounces shredded nonfat mozzarella-style soy cheese or part-skim or nonfat mozzarella cheese (¾ cup)

2 tablespoons shredded or grated Parmesan cheese

Heat a large skillet over medium-high heat. Remove from heat and spray with vegetable oil spray. Cook mushrooms, zucchini, and onions for 8 minutes, or until zucchini is tender, stirring frequently.

Meanwhile, in a medium bowl, whisk together egg substitute, milk, parsley, oregano, and salt.

Stir pasta into vegetables; pour egg mixture over all. Reduce heat to medium-low and cook, covered, for 8 minutes.

Sprinkle with mozzarella. Remove from heat and let stand, covered, for 5 minutes to continue cooking and melt cheese.

Sprinkle with Parmesan. Cut into six wedges.

CAJUN FRITTATA WITH PASTA

Substitute chopped green or red bell pepper for zucchini, Cajun seasoning for salt, and 3 ounces shredded reduced-fat or fat-free sharp Cheddar cheese for mozzarella and Parmesan. (Calories 155; Protein 12 g; Carbohydrates 20 g; Cholesterol 9 mg; Total Fat 3 g; Saturated 1 g; Polyunsaturated 0 g; Monounsaturated 1 g; Fiber 2 g; Sodium 210 mg)

COOK'S TIP

If you don't have any leftover cooked pasta, cook 4 ounces dried angel hair pasta while cooking vegetables. Use package directions, but omit salt and oil. Don't use fresh pasta in this recipe. It will break down and become a solid mass.

(PER SERVING)

Calories 139

Protein 12 g

Carbohydrates 20 g

Cholesterol 2 mg

Total Fat 1 g

  Saturated 1 g

  Polyunsaturated 0 g

  Monounsaturated 0 g

Fiber 2 g

Sodium 329 mg

Italian Gnocchi with Vegetables

- Serves 4; 1 heaping cup per serving
- Preparation time: 5 minutes
- Cooking time: 22 to 24 minutes

Who can resist plump potato dumplings, known as gnocchi (NYO-kee), especially when they are bathed in an Italian-flavored sauce with carrots, tomatoes, and spinach?

8 cups water

1 teaspoon olive oil

½ to 1 cup frozen chopped onion or 1 medium to large onion, thinly sliced

1 teaspoon bottled minced garlic or 2 medium cloves garlic, minced

14.5-ounce can no-salt-added crushed tomatoes

½ teaspoon fennel seeds (optional)

½ teaspoon sugar

¼ teaspoon salt

⅛ teaspoon pepper

½ to ¾ cup baby carrots

9-ounce package frozen no-salt-added artichoke hearts

8 ounces gnocchi or any uncooked pasta

6 ounces baby spinach leaves

2 teaspoons fresh rosemary, chopped, or ½ teaspoon dried, crushed

Pour water into a large saucepan or stockpot. Cover and bring to a boil over high heat.

Meanwhile, heat a large skillet over medium-high heat. Add olive oil and swirl to coat bottom of skillet. Cook onion and garlic for 2 to 3 minutes, or until onion is tender, stirring occasionally.

Stir tomatoes, fennel seeds, sugar, salt, and pepper into onion mixture (if using dried rosemary, add here); bring to a simmer over medium-high heat. Reduce heat and simmer, uncovered, for 6 to 8 minutes, stirring occasionally.

When water is boiling, add carrots to pan; reduce heat to medium-high and cook for 2 to 3 minutes.

Add artichokes and gnocchi to carrots; bring to a boil over high heat. Reduce heat to medium-high and cook for 6 minutes, or until tender.

Add spinach to carrot mixture and cook for 1 to 2 minutes. Drain in a colander, then stir into tomato mixture.

Add fresh rosemary. Reduce heat to low and cook for 1 to 2 minutes, or until mixture is warmed through.

GNOCCHI WITH ITALIAN TURKEY SAUSAGE AND VEGETABLES

While water comes to a boil, remove casings from 3 ounces low-fat Italian turkey sausage. In a large nonstick skillet, cook sausage over medium-high heat for 4 to 5 minutes, or until no longer pink in center, stirring to break up sausage. Put in a colander and rinse with hot water to remove excess fat; drain well. Wipe skillet with paper towels. Set sausage aside and continue with above recipe, omitting fennel seeds (sauté vegetables in the skillet used for sausage). Add sausage with tomatoes and continue with recipe. Serves 4; 1¼ cups per serving. (Calories 248; Protein 11 g; Carbohydrates 45 g; Cholesterol 8 mg; Total Fat 3 g; Saturated 1 g; Polyunsaturated 1 g; Monounsaturated 1 g; Fiber 9 g; Sodium 389 mg)

COOK'S TIP ON GNOCCHI

Look in the pasta section (though they aren't pasta) or the gourmet section of the grocery store for gnocchi. They're vacuum-packed, then boxed. Refrigerate leftover uncooked gnocchi for several days; freeze for longer storage.

(PER SERVING)

Calories 222
Protein 7 g
Carbohydrates 44 g
Cholesterol 0 mg
Total Fat 2 g
  Saturated 0 g
  Polyunsaturated 0 g
  Monounsaturated 1 g
Fiber 9 g
Sodium 272 mg

Mozzarella Polenta with Roasted Vegetable Salsa

- Serves 4; 2 polenta rounds and ½ cup salsa per serving
- Preparation time: 15 minutes
- Cooking time: 14 minutes

This vegetable-rich entrée is a breeze to make with prepared polenta.

Vegetable oil spray

16-ounce package prepared fat-free polenta

Salsa

2 medium tomatoes (10 to 12 ounces)

1 large green bell pepper (about 8 ounces)

1 large zucchini (about 8 ounces) (optional)

1 large crookneck squash (about 7 ounces)

Vegetable oil spray

1 tablespoon cider vinegar

2 teaspoons extra-virgin olive oil

1 teaspoon dried oregano, crumbled

½ teaspoon bottled minced garlic or 1 medium clove garlic, minced

⅛ teaspoon salt

¼ cup finely snipped fresh parsley or fresh cilantro

■ ■ ■

2 ounces (½ cup) shredded nonfat or part-skim mozzarella cheese

Preheat broiler. Line two baking sheets with aluminum foil. Spray foil with vegetable oil spray.

Gently rinse polenta under running water; pat dry with paper towels. Cut polenta into eight rounds, put on one baking sheet, and set aside.

For salsa, cut tomatoes in half crosswise and put cut side up on second baking sheet. Cut pepper in half lengthwise and remove ribs, seeds, and stem. Flatten each half with palm, pulling out any parts of pepper that curve under; put on same baking sheet. Cut zucchini and crookneck squash in half lengthwise and add cut side up to baking sheet. Lightly spray vegetables with vegetable oil spray.

Broil for 5 minutes about 4 inches from heat. Turn vegetables over and broil for 3 minutes, or until lightly charred.

Meanwhile, in a small bowl, stir together remaining salsa ingredients except parsley; set aside.

Using a knife and fork, coarsely chop vegetables. In a medium mixing bowl, stir together vegetables, vinegar mixture, and parsley. Cover with aluminum foil to keep warm.

Broil polenta for 3 minutes, turn rounds over, and broil for 2 minutes. Sprinkle with mozzarella and broil for 1 minute, or until beginning to lightly brown.

To serve, arrange two polenta rounds on each of four dinner plates; then spoon about ½ cup salsa mixture on and around polenta.

COOK'S TIP

The salsa is also delicious served at room temperature. For peak flavor, wait until serving time to toss vegetables with vinegar mixture.

COOK'S TIP ON POLENTA

Look for prepared polenta (basically cornmeal cooked with water) in plastic-wrapped cylinders, usually in the produce department. Because it doesn't need refrigeration, it may be with the pastas instead. In addition to plain polenta, you'll also discover everything from Mexican-inspired combinations to polenta flavored with wild mushrooms.

(PER SERVING)

Calories 166

Protein 8 g

Carbohydrates 26 g

Cholesterol 3 mg

Total Fat 3 g

  Saturated 0 g

  Polyunsaturated 0 g

  Monounsaturated 2 g

Fiber 5 g

Sodium 429 mg

Mushroom Quesadillas

- Serves 4; 3 pieces per serving
- Preparation time: 10 minutes
- Cooking time: 8 minutes
- Microwave time: 1 minute

Mushrooms and chiles are covered with cheese that's been fired with jalapeño, then wrapped in a warm tortilla to make a rich and creamy Tex-Mex treat.

13¼-ounce can sliced mushrooms, drained

½ cup reduced-fat cream of mushroom soup

2 tablespoons chopped canned green chiles, rinsed and drained

Vegetable oil spray

4 6-inch corn tortillas

¾ to 1 cup grated reduced-fat jalapeño Jack or Monterey Jack cheese

¼ cup spicy salsa

In a medium saucepan, combine mushrooms, soup, and chiles. Cook over medium heat for 2 minutes, or until heated through, stirring occasionally.

Meanwhile, heat a griddle or large skillet over medium-high heat. Remove it from heat and spray with vegetable oil spray. Warm 1 tortilla for about 1 minute on each side, or until it softens. Repeat with remaining tortillas.

To assemble, place warm tortillas on a microwave-safe tray. Spread filling on one half of each tortilla, leaving ½ inch around edge. Sprinkle cheese over filling. Fold each tortilla in half over filling. Press edges together.

Microwave on 100 percent power (high) for 1 minute.

To serve, cut each tortilla into three pieces. Put a dab of salsa on each piece.

(PER SERVING)

Calories 186

Protein 11 g

Carbohydrates 22 g

Cholesterol 18 mg

Total Fat 6 g

  Saturated 3 g

  Polyunsaturated —

  Monounsaturated —

Fiber 4 g

Sodium 375 mg

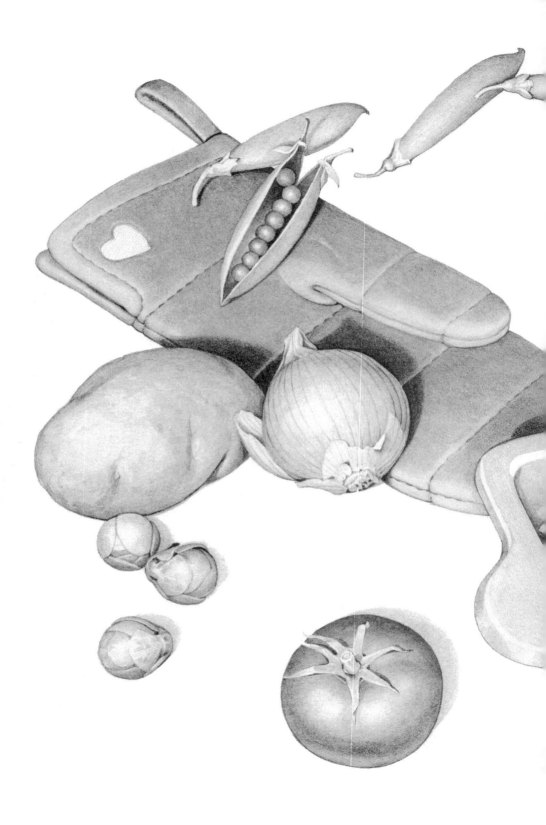

VEGETABLES
AND SIDE DISHES

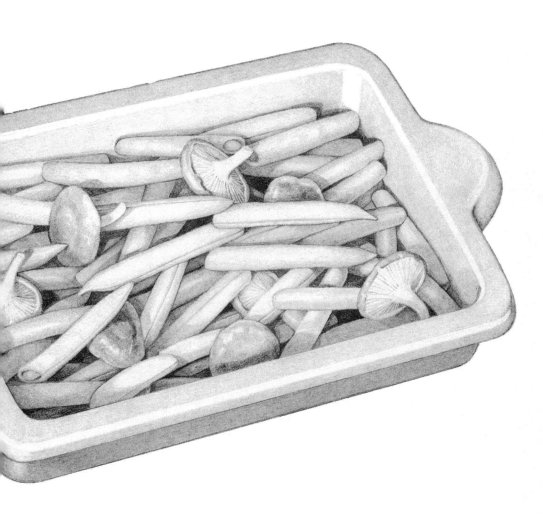

■ ■ ■

Roasted, Toasted Asparagus

Broccoli with Sweet-and-Sour
Tangerine Sauce

Sesame Broccoli

Curried Brussels Sprouts

Maple-Glazed Carrots

Black-Peppered Corn

Greek Green Beans

Mixed Mushrooms and Spinach

Herbed Peas and Mushrooms

Bell Peppers with Nuts
and Olives

Roasted Red and White Potatoes

Coconut-Scented Rice
with Almonds

Savory Pecan Rice

Creamed Spinach

Creamed Peas

Orange-Flavored Acorn Squash
and Sweet Potato

Bulgur-Stuffed Crookneck Squash

■ ■ ■

Roasted, Toasted Asparagus

Serves 4; 4 ounces per serving ■
Preparation time: 10 minutes ■
Cooking time: 4 minutes ■

Roasting the asparagus intensifies its natural flavor and sweetness, and the toasted sesame oil adds a subtle nuttiness. You can serve this dish warm or at room temperature, which makes it a natural for a buffet.

Vegetable oil spray

1 pound fresh asparagus (16 to 20 medium spears)

2 teaspoons toasted sesame oil

⅛ teaspoon salt

Preheat broiler. Line a baking sheet with aluminum foil. Spray foil with vegetable oil spray.

Trim about 1 inch from bottom of asparagus. Dry thoroughly with paper towels. Place asparagus in a single layer on baking sheet. Lightly spray asparagus with vegetable oil spray.

Broil about 4 inches from heat for 4 minutes, or just until asparagus is tender-crisp and a few brown spots appear. Remove from broiler.

Using a pastry brush, brush sesame oil over asparagus and sprinkle with salt.

Cook's Tip on Asparagus

To trim asparagus, hold the cut end of a spear. Bend it gently until you feel where the tough part of the spear begins, often about 1 inch from the bottom. Snap the spear at that point, discarding the tough end. A rule of thumb is that the thinner the asparagus, the tenderer it will be. If you peel the thicker stalks, they'll also be tender.

(PER SERVING)

Calories 32
Protein 1 g
Carbohydrates 2 g
Cholesterol 0 mg
Total Fat 2 g
  Saturated 0 g
  Polyunsaturated —
  Monounsaturated —
Fiber 1 g
Sodium 77 mg

Broccoli with Sweet-and-Sour Tangerine Sauce

- Serves 4; ½ cup broccoli and 1 tablespoon sauce per serving
- Preparation time: 10 minutes
- Cooking time: 8 to 11 minutes

This sweet-and-sour side dish pairs nicely with Asian recipes, as well as with ham or turkey. On its own, the sauce enhances almost any cooked vegetable or meat and is good as a dipping sauce for Turkey Potstickers (pages 44–45).

2 cups broccoli florets (about 8 ounces)

Tangerine Sauce

¼ cup tangerine or orange marmalade

1 to 2 tablespoons rice vinegar

½ teaspoon grated gingerroot or ⅛ teaspoon ground ginger

2 to 3 drops hot pepper oil

Put broccoli in a steamer basket in a medium saucepan over a small amount of simmering water. Cook, covered, for 6 to 8 minutes, or until tender.

Meanwhile, in a small saucepan, stir together sauce ingredients. Cook over low heat for 2 to 3 minutes, or until marmalade has melted, stirring occasionally.

To serve, spoon about 1 tablespoon sauce onto each plate and place broccoli on top.

(PER SERVING)

Calories 65

Protein 1 g

Carbohydrates 16 g

Cholesterol 0 mg

Total Fat 0 g

  Saturated 0 g

  Polyunsaturated 0 g

  Monounsaturated 0 g

Fiber 1 g

Sodium 15 mg

Sesame Broccoli

Serves 4; ½ cup per serving ■
Preparation time: 10 minutes ■
Cooking time: 10 minutes ■

The rich-tasting sesame seeds add lots of flavor to this dish. If you use the broccoli stems, you can serve six people.

1 head broccoli

1 teaspoon olive or other acceptable vegetable oil

1 tablespoon sesame seeds

2 tablespoons water

1 tablespoon light soy sauce

⅛ to ¼ teaspoon crushed red pepper flakes

1½ teaspoons lemon juice

Cut broccoli into small florets. If desired, peel and dice stems and add to florets.

In a large skillet, heat oil over medium-high heat. Cook sesame seeds for 1 minute, stirring constantly.

Add broccoli and cook over high heat until it turns bright green, about 3 minutes, stirring constantly.

Stir in remaining ingredients. Reduce heat to medium and cook, covered, for 5 minutes, or until broccoli is desired texture.

(PER SERVING)

Calories 50

Protein 3 g

Carbohydrates 5 g

Cholesterol 1 mg

Total Fat 3 g

  Saturated 0 g

  Polyunsaturated 0 g

  Monounsaturated 1 g

Fiber 3 g

Sodium 122 mg

Curried Brussels Sprouts

- Serves 4; ½ cup per serving
- Preparation time: 10 minutes
- Cooking time: 25 minutes

Curry powder and creamy sauce turn brussels sprouts into company fare.

½ cup water

¼ cup frozen chopped onion or ½ medium onion (sweet preferred)

10-ounce package frozen no-salt-added brussels sprouts

2 teaspoons cornstarch

1 cup low-sodium chicken broth (divided use)

⅛ teaspoon curry powder or ½ teaspoon mild curry paste

⅛ teaspoon white pepper

2 tablespoons shredded or grated Parmesan cheese

Preheat oven to 350° F.

In a medium saucepan, bring water to a boil over high heat.

Meanwhile, if using fresh onion, cut into 1-inch pieces. Add onion and brussels sprouts to saucepan; return to a boil. Reduce heat and simmer, covered, for 4 minutes; drain.

While sprouts simmer, put cornstarch in a small saucepan. Add ¼ cup broth and whisk together until cornstarch is dissolved. Whisk in remaining broth; bring to a boil over medium heat. Cook for 1 minute, or until mixture bubbles, stirring once or twice. (Sauce will be a little thicker than a thin cream sauce.)

Stir in curry powder and pepper, then combine with drained vegetables. Pour into a 1-quart casserole dish and sprinkle with Parmesan.

Bake for 15 minutes, or until bubbly and slightly browned.

(PER SERVING)

Calories 62

Protein 5 g

Carbohydrates 9 g

Cholesterol 2 mg

Total Fat 2 g

Saturated 1 g

Polyunsaturated 0 g

Monounsaturated 0 g

Fiber 3 g

Sodium 90 mg

Maple-Glazed Carrots

Serves 4; ½ cup per serving ■
Preparation time: 5 minutes ■
Cooking time: 12 to 15 minutes ■

Looking for a way to get the kids to eat their carrots? Baby carrots with maple syrup and cinnamon are practically dessert!

½ cup water

1 pound baby carrots, or whole carrots cut into ⅛-inch diagonal slices

3 tablespoons maple syrup or pancake syrup

1 tablespoon acceptable margarine

¼ teaspoon ground cinnamon

In a large nonstick skillet, bring water to a boil over high heat; add carrots. Reduce heat and simmer, covered, for 8 minutes, or until just tender-crisp. Drain well on paper towels and pat dry. Dry skillet with a paper towel, if necessary. Return carrots to skillet.

Stir remaining ingredients into skillet. Bring to a boil over high heat; cook for 2 to 3 minutes, or until richly glazed, stirring constantly. Serve immediately.

COOK'S TIP

The secret to achieving a rich glaze is to dry the carrots thoroughly before adding the other ingredients. For peak flavor and to have a glazed effect, it's important to serve this dish immediately. You can, however, cook the carrots and assemble the glaze ingredients ahead of time.

(PER SERVING)

Calories 106

Protein 1 g

Carbohydrates 19 g

Cholesterol 0 mg

Total Fat 3 g

  Saturated 1 g

  Polyunsaturated 1 g

  Monounsaturated 1 g

Fiber 3 g

Sodium 75 mg

Black-Peppered Corn

- Serves 4; ½ cup per serving
- Preparation time: 5 minutes
- Cooking time: 7 minutes

Lightly browning the margarine gives this corn dish a nutty taste.

16-ounce package frozen no-salt-
  added whole-kernel corn, thawed

Vegetable oil spray

2 teaspoons acceptable margarine

¼ teaspoon salt

⅛ to ¼ teaspoon black pepper

⅛ teaspoon paprika

3 tablespoons water

Pat corn dry with paper towels.

Heat a large nonstick skillet over high heat. Remove skillet from heat and spray with vegetable oil spray. Add margarine and swirl to coat bottom of skillet. Heat until margarine begins to brown, about 30 seconds.

Add corn and cook until browned, about 3 minutes, stirring constantly.

Stir in remaining ingredients except water; cook for 30 seconds, stirring constantly.

Add water and scrape bottom of skillet with flat spatula to loosen any particles. Stir and serve.

(PER SERVING)

Calories 117

Protein 3 g

Carbohydrates 24 g

Cholesterol 0 mg

Total Fat 3 g

  Saturated 0 g

  Polyunsaturated 1 g

  Monounsaturated 1 g

Fiber 3 g

Sodium 172 mg

Greek Green Beans

Serves 8; ½ cup per serving ■
Preparation time: 15 minutes ■
Cooking time: 18 to 23 minutes ■

Pairing green beans and tomatoes makes great sense in the summertime when both are fresh in the garden or at farmers' markets. Use fresh beans and tomatoes if you have them and have the time. Substitute frozen beans and canned tomatoes if you're rushed.

1 pound fresh or frozen no-salt-added green beans

2 teaspoons olive oil

½ cup frozen chopped onion or 1 medium onion, chopped

⅛ teaspoon crushed red pepper flakes, or to taste

¼ cup water (plus more as needed)

½ teaspoon dried dillweed, crumbled

¼ teaspoon salt

¼ teaspoon freshly ground pepper, or to taste

3 medium tomatoes, minced, or 14.5-ounce can no-salt-added crushed tomatoes

2 ounces feta cheese, rinsed and crumbled

Trim green beans if using fresh.

Heat a wide, deep skillet over medium-high heat. Add oil and swirl to coat bottom of skillet. Cook onion and red pepper flakes for 2 minutes, or until onions are translucent, stirring occasionally.

Add green beans, water, dillweed, salt, and pepper. Cook for 10 to 15 minutes, or until beans are almost cooked to taste, adding water if necessary.

Add tomatoes and cook for 2 to 5 minutes, or until beans are cooked to taste (fresh green beans will take a little longer to cook than frozen).

To serve, sprinkle with feta.

Cook's Tip

To reduce the amount of sodium, total fat, and saturated fat in this dish, you can omit the feta. You'll lose 60 milligrams of sodium, the fat will decrease by 2 grams, and the saturated fat will fall to 0 grams.

(PER SERVING)

Calories 56
Protein 2 g
Carbohydrates 7 g
Cholesterol 6 mg
Total Fat 3 g
  Saturated 1 g
  Polyunsaturated 0 g
  Monounsaturated 2 g
Fiber 2 g
Sodium 141 mg

Mixed Mushrooms and Spinach

- Serves 4; ½ cup per serving
- Preparation time: 10 minutes
- Soaking time: 10 minutes
- Cooking time: 7 minutes

This richly flavored vegetable mixture enhances simple beef or chicken dishes. For a lively light entrée, serve the vegetables over rice.

3 tablespoons dried mushrooms
  (porcini preferred)
¼ cup hot water
5 cups fresh spinach (about 8 ounces)
¼ cup low-sodium chicken broth
10 ounces presliced fresh mushrooms

¼ teaspoon salt (optional)
Freshly ground black pepper
2 tablespoons dry sherry
¼ teaspoon ground nutmeg
⅛ teaspoon crushed red pepper flakes
  (optional)

(PER SERVING)
Calories 58
Protein 4 g
Carbohydrates 10 g
Cholesterol 0 mg
Total Fat 1 g
  Saturated 0 g
  Polyunsaturated 0 g
  Monounsaturated 0 g
Fiber 3 g
Sodium 67 mg

In a small bowl, soak dried mushrooms in hot water and let sit for 10 minutes.

Meanwhile, coarsely chop spinach; set aside.

In a large skillet, bring broth to a simmer over medium-high heat. Sauté fresh mushrooms for about 2 minutes, or until they begin to give off their liquid, stirring frequently.

Add salt, black pepper, and sherry; slightly increase heat. Cook for about 3 minutes, or until liquid is slightly reduced.

Drain and chop dried mushrooms, reserving 1 tablespoon liquid. Add chopped mushrooms, reserved liquid, and spinach to mushroom mixture in skillet. Cook over medium heat for about 1 minute, or until spinach is just wilted, stirring constantly.

Stir in nutmeg and red pepper.

COOK'S TIP ON MUSHROOMS

Fresh mushrooms readily absorb water, so don't soak them or rinse them to clean off the surface dirt. Instead, brush them lightly with a damp paper towel or a mushroom brush.

Herbed Peas and Mushrooms

Serves 6; ¾ cup per serving ■
Preparation time: 5 minutes ■
Cooking time: 9 to 12 minutes ■

As an accompaniment for anything from roasted turkey at a holiday feast to grilled burgers on the patio, this side dish is hard to beat.

1 teaspoon extra-virgin olive oil

10 ounces presliced fresh mushrooms (button, cremini, portobello, or a combination)

1 large onion, coarsely chopped (sweet preferred) (about ¾ cup)

16-ounce package frozen tiny or regular-size green peas (about 3 cups)

¼ cup orange juice

½ teaspoon dried mint, crumbled

¼ to ½ teaspoon dried oregano, crumbled

⅛ to ¼ teaspoon pepper

Heat a large skillet over medium heat. Add oil and swirl to coat bottom of skillet. Cook mushrooms and onion, covered, for 7 to 9 minutes, or until mushrooms are tender, stirring occasionally.

Stir in remaining ingredients. Cook, covered, for 2 to 3 minutes, or until heated through, stirring occasionally.

(PER SERVING)

Calories 91

Protein 5 g

Carbohydrates 16 g

Cholesterol 0 mg

Total Fat 1 g

  Saturated 0 g

  Polyunsaturated 0 g

  Monounsaturated 1 g

Fiber 5 g

Sodium 88 mg

Bell Peppers with Nuts and Olives

- Serves 8; ⅔ cup per serving
- Preparation time: 10 minutes
- Cooking time: 10 to 15 minutes

Nuts and olives make this an extra-fancy side dish to serve with baked chicken or on a vegetable plate. You can make a simpler dish by eliminating those condiments, however.

2 tablespoons pine nuts or chopped pecans

3 medium bell peppers (various colors) or 2 1-pound bags frozen mixed bell pepper strips or frozen bell peppers with onions

1 medium onion (omit if using frozen bell pepper and onion combination)

1 tablespoon olive oil

1 teaspoon bottled minced garlic or 2 medium cloves garlic, minced

⅛ to ¼ teaspoon salt

⅛ to ¼ teaspoon freshly ground pepper, or to taste

2 tablespoons chopped imported black or stuffed green olives

In a large skillet, dry-roast nuts over medium heat for 1 to 5 minutes, or until they're aromatic and turning golden, stirring frequently. Transfer to a small dish.

Meanwhile, remove and discard core, seeds, and stems from bell peppers; slice peppers and onion.

Add olive oil to same skillet and swirl to coat bottom. Increase heat to high. Cook bell peppers, onion, and garlic, stirring occasionally, for about 5 minutes if peppers are frozen, 10 to 15 minutes if fresh, or until desired tenderness—preferably not too limp.

Stir in salt and pepper.

To serve, transfer to a platter or individual plates and sprinkle with olives and nuts.

COOK'S TIP ON SKILLETS

A heavy skillet heats more evenly and cooks food more quickly. Thinner skillets tend to burn in some areas while undercooking in others.

(PER SERVING)

Calories 43

Protein 1 g

Carbohydrates 4 g

Cholesterol 0 mg

Total Fat 3 g

  Saturated 0 g

  Polyunsaturated 1 g

  Monounsaturated 2 g

Fiber 1 g

Sodium 93 mg

Roasted Red and White Potatoes

Serves 6; ½ cup per serving (plus 3 cups reserved) ∎
Preparation time: 10 minutes ∎
Cooking time: 40 minutes ∎

One kind of roasted potato is good, and two kinds are doubly delicious. This recipe is twice as good in another way too. You get roasted potatoes for today and a start on German or Mexican Potato Salad for later (page 79).

Olive oil spray

2½ pounds small potatoes, red and white

1 tablespoon chopped fresh rosemary or 1 teaspoon dried, crushed

2 teaspoons olive oil

¼ to ½ teaspoon salt

Freshly ground pepper to taste

1 large onion (sweet preferred)

Preheat oven to 425° F. Spray a jelly-roll pan with olive oil spray.

Cut potatoes into 1-inch cubes and pat dry with paper towels. In a large bowl, combine potatoes with remaining ingredients except onion. Spread in a single layer in prepared pan.

Roast for 20 minutes, stirring after 10 minutes.

Meanwhile, cut onion into 1-inch cubes.

After potatoes have cooked for 20 minutes, add onions, stirring well. Roast for 20 minutes, or until potatoes are lightly browned and tender when pierced with a fork, stirring after 10 minutes.

Cook's Tip

If onions seem to be browning too quickly, stir more frequently.

(PER SERVING)

Calories 94

Protein 2 g

Carbohydrates 20 g

Cholesterol 0 mg

Total Fat 1 g

   Saturated 0 g

   Polyunsaturated 0 g

   Monounsaturated 1 g

Fiber 2 g

Sodium 77 mg

Coconut-Scented Rice with Almonds

- Serves 8; ½ cup per serving
- Preparation time: 5 minutes
- Cooking time: 21 to 22 minutes

Using a small amount of crushed toasted almonds lets you distribute their nutty flavor throughout this dish without adding much fat.

2 cups fat-free milk

¼ teaspoon salt

2 cups uncooked instant rice

1 ounce sliced almonds (¼ to ⅓ cup)

½ teaspoon coconut extract

In a medium saucepan, bring milk and salt to a boil over medium-high heat, about 12 minutes.

Stir in rice; return to a boil, about 1 minute. Reduce heat and simmer, covered, for 5 to 6 minutes, or until liquid is absorbed.

Meanwhile, heat a large nonstick skillet over medium heat. Dry-roast almonds until richly golden brown and fragrant, 1 to 5 minutes, stirring frequently. Transfer to a small plate and let cool for 1 minute. Using back of a spoon or fork, finely crush almonds. Or put almonds in a plastic bag or wrap loosely in plastic wrap and crush with a rolling pin or side of a glass.

Add extract to rice, fluff with a fork, and stir in almonds.

(PER SERVING)

Calories 132

Protein 5 g

Carbohydrates 24 g

Cholesterol 1 mg

Total Fat 2 g

  Saturated 0 g

  Polyunsaturated 0 g

  Monounsaturated 1 g

Fiber 1 g

Sodium 107 mg

Savory Pecan Rice

Serves 6; ¼ cup per serving ■
Preparation time: 5 minutes ■
Cooking time: 23 to 25 minutes ■

With their assertive flavors, the dried fruit, nuts, and mushrooms in this dish pair well with poultry or game. You can also use this recipe to make a vegetarian stuffing for baked winter squash, such as butternut.

2 cups water

7-ounce package pecan rice or 1 cup other uncooked aromatic rice

¼ cup dried cherries (about 1 ounce)

½ teaspoon salt

1 teaspoon olive oil

8 ounces presliced fresh mushrooms

½ large red bell pepper, chopped (about ½ cup)

½ teaspoon fennel seeds or 1 teaspoon dried thyme, crumbled

¼ cup chopped pecans (about 1 ounce)

In a large saucepan, combine water, rice, cherries, and salt; bring to a boil over high heat, 3 to 5 minutes. Reduce heat to low and cook, covered, for 20 minutes, or until rice is tender.

Meanwhile, heat a large nonstick skillet over high heat. Add oil and swirl to coat bottom of skillet. Cook mushrooms, bell pepper, and fennel seeds for about 7 minutes, or until bell pepper is soft, stirring occasionally. Transfer to a medium-size serving bowl.

Stir in pecans and rice.

(PER SERVING)

Calories 176

Protein 4 g

Carbohydrates 31 g

Cholesterol 0 mg

Total Fat 5 g

  Saturated 0 g

  Polyunsaturated 1 g

  Monounsaturated 2 g

Fiber 2 g

Sodium 207 mg

Creamed Spinach

- Serves 8; ½ cup per serving
- Preparation time: 5 minutes
- Cooking time: 10 to 12 minutes

Serve this creamy side dish with crispy oven-baked fish or chicken. Since the recipe makes a lot, you may want to use part of the mixture over cooked pasta or brown rice later in the week.

2 10-ounce packages frozen chopped spinach

2 cups fat-free milk

10.5-ounce can reduced-fat, reduced-sodium cream of chicken soup

1 teaspoon very low sodium or low-sodium Worcestershire sauce

¼ teaspoon pepper

In a medium saucepan, cook spinach using package directions, omitting salt and margarine. Drain well and squeeze out as much moisture as possible. Return spinach to saucepan.

Stir in remaining ingredients. Cook over medium heat for 7 to 8 minutes, or until mixture is heated through, stirring occasionally.

CREAMED PEAS

Substitute 4 cups frozen peas for spinach, and reduce milk to 1 cup. Combine all ingredients (no need to thaw peas) in a medium saucepan. Cook over medium heat for 8 to 10 minutes, or until peas are tender and mixture is heated through, stirring occasionally. Serves 8; ½ cup per serving. (Calories 89; Protein 5 g; Carbohydrates 15 g; Cholesterol 5 mg; Total Fat 1 g; Saturated 0 g; Polyunsaturated 0 g; Monounsaturated 0 g; Fiber 3 g; Sodium 248 mg)

(PER SERVING)

Calories 61

Protein 5 g

Carbohydrates 10 g

Cholesterol 6 mg

Total Fat 1 g

Saturated 1 g

Polyunsaturated 0 g

Monounsaturated 0 g

Fiber 2 g

Sodium 235 mg

Orange-Flavored Acorn Squash and Sweet Potato

Serves 6 ∎

Preparation time: 20 minutes ∎

Cooking time: 30 minutes ∎

Serve this decorative side dish with your holiday meal or with roast beef for Sunday dinner. Baking at a high temperature slightly caramelizes the bottom of the squash for a delightful taste.

Vegetable oil spray

1 teaspoon orange zest

2 tablespoons orange juice

2 teaspoons light margarine, melted

1 medium acorn squash (about 1½ pounds)

6- to 8-ounce sweet potato

2 tablespoons light brown sugar

¼ teaspoon ground mace or nutmeg

Vegetable oil spray

Preheat oven to 400° F. Spray one extra-large or two large nonstick baking pans with vegetable oil spray; set aside.

In a small bowl, stir together orange zest, orange juice, and margarine; set aside.

Trim ends of squash. Cut crosswise into ¼-inch slices (about 12 slices). Using a spoon, remove seeds. Peel sweet potato and cut into ⅛-inch slices.

To assemble, put squash slices in one layer on baking sheet(s). Place 4 or 5 overlapping slices of sweet potato in center of each squash ring. Pour a small amount of orange juice mixture over each stack. Sprinkle with brown sugar and mace, then lightly spray with vegetable oil spray.

Bake for 30 minutes, or until vegetables are tender when pierced with a fork. Use a large, flat spatula to remove slices.

(PER SERVING)

Calories 76

Protein 1 g

Carbohydrates 19 g

Cholesterol 0 mg

Total Fat 0 g

  Saturated 0 g

   Polyunsaturated 0 g

   Monounsaturated 0 g

Fiber 2 g

Sodium 8 mg

Bulgur-Stuffed Crookneck Squash

- Serves 8; 1 piece per serving
- Preparation time: 10 minutes
- Cooking time: 29 to 33 minutes

An attractive dish for entertaining, this recipe has a Middle Eastern flavor. If you are really in a hurry, try the alternate cooking method. It's an Express-ipe, taking only 25 minutes, start to finish.

4 medium crookneck squash
   (1¼ to 1½ pounds)

2 tablespoons water

½ cup whole fresh mushrooms, stems removed

1 teaspoon olive oil

¼ cup frozen chopped onion or ½ medium onion, chopped

½ cup frozen peas

½ cup low-sodium chicken broth

¼ cup roasted red bell peppers, rinsed, drained, and chopped (optional)

¼ cup bulgur wheat

½ teaspoon dried dillweed, crumbled

⅛ teaspoon black pepper

1 tablespoon plus 1 teaspoon shredded or grated Parmesan cheese

1 tablespoon plus 1 teaspoon pine nuts

Preheat oven to 350° F.

Cut squash in half lengthwise. Use a spoon or melon baller to scoop out pulp, leaving eight shells (reserve pulp).

Put squash cut side down in a 13 x 9 x 2-inch nonstick baking pan; pour water into pan.

Bake, uncovered, for 8 to 10 minutes, or until squash is tender. Drain liquid and turn squash over. Leave oven on.

Meanwhile, process pulp and mushrooms in a food processor or blender for 10 to 15 seconds, or until coarsely chopped.

Heat a large skillet over medium-high heat. Add oil and swirl to coat bottom of skillet. Cook squash mixture and onion for 2 minutes, or until onion is translucent, stirring occasionally.

Add peas, broth, roasted peppers, bulgur, dillweed, and black pepper; bring to a simmer over medium-high heat. Reduce heat to medium-low and cook, covered, for 10 minutes, or until bulgur is tender. Spoon into reserved squash shells.

Sprinkle squash with Parmesan and pine nuts.

Bake for 6 to 8 minutes, or until warmed through.

Alternate Cooking Method

Thinly slice squash and mushrooms. Cook as directed above with olive oil and onion. Add peas, broth, roasted peppers, bulgur, dillweed, and black pepper. Bring to a boil over high heat; reduce heat to medium-low and cook, covered, for 10 minutes, as directed above. Sprinkle with Parmesan and pine nuts. (No baking needed.) Makes eight ½-cup servings.

(PER SERVING)

Calories 63

Protein 3 g

Carbohydrates 9 g

Cholesterol 1 mg

Total Fat 2 g

Saturated 0 g

Polyunsaturated 0 g

Monounsaturated 1 g

Fiber 2 g

Sodium 36 mg

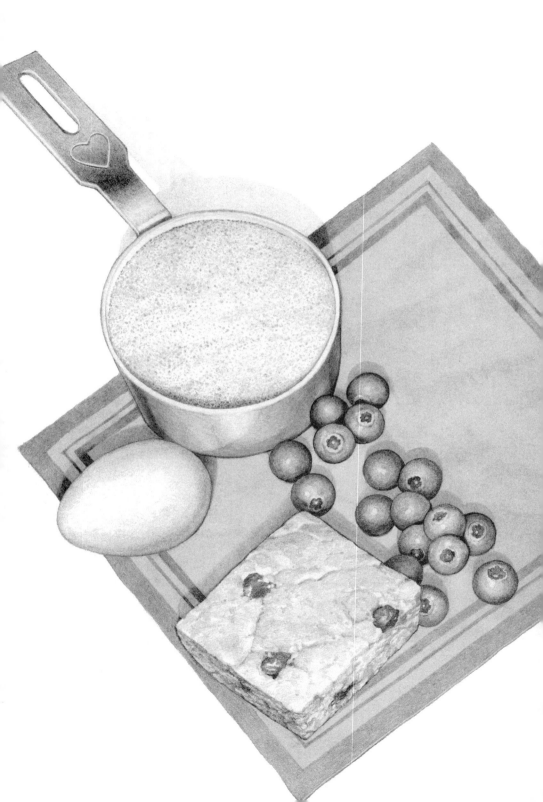

BREADS AND
BREAKFAST DISHES

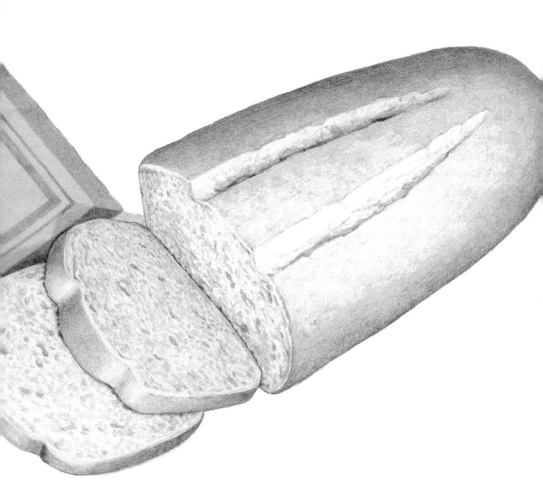

■ ■ ■

Herb Sticks

    Cinnamon Sticks

Lemony Blueberry Coffeecake

    Raspberry Coffeecake

Mini Cinnamon Stackups

Yogurt Brûlée with Blueberries

Fruitful Brown Rice Cereal

Huevos Rancheros Casserole

■ ■ ■

Herb Sticks

Serves 5; 3 sticks per serving ■
Preparation time: 5 minutes ■
Cooking time: 8 minutes ■

Serve these garlicky bread sticks with Cheddar Jack Chili Mac (page 209).

Vegetable oil spray

7-ounce package refrigerated low-fat soft bread sticks

Vegetable oil spray (plain, butter, or olive oil variety)

½ teaspoon salt-free garlic-flavored Italian seasoning

1 tablespoon plus 1½ teaspoons shredded or grated Parmesan cheese

Preheat oven to 400° F. Spray a nonstick baking sheet with vegetable oil spray.

Carefully unroll and separate bread dough. Cut each stick of dough into thirds so that each new bread stick measures about 4 inches long. Put on baking sheet. Lightly spray bread sticks with vegetable oil spray and sprinkle with seasoning mixture.

Bake for 8 to 10 minutes, or until golden brown. Remove from oven and sprinkle with Parmesan. Serve immediately.

CINNAMON STICKS

Use plain or butter-flavor vegetable oil spray. Replace Italian seasoning and Parmesan cheese with a mixture of 1 tablespoon plus 1½ teaspoons sugar and 1 teaspoon ground cinnamon. (Calories 130; Protein 3 g; Carbohydrates 23 g; Cholesterol 0 mg; Total Fat 2 g; Saturated 1 g; Polyunsaturated —; Monounsaturated —; Fiber 1 g; Sodium 289 mg)

(PER SERVING)

Calories 122
Protein 4 g
Carbohydrates 19 g
Cholesterol 1 mg
Total Fat 2 g
   Saturated 1 g
    Polyunsaturated —
    Monounsaturated —
Fiber 0 g
Sodium 318 mg

BREADS AND BREAKFAST DISHES

Lemony Blueberry Coffeecake

- Serves 15; 2½ x 3-inch slice per serving
- Preparation time: 20 minutes
- Cooking time: 30 to 38 minutes
- Cooling time: 10 to 20 minutes

Serve this delicately flavored moist cake warm from the oven for brunch. If there is any left over, pack it in lunches or serve it for dessert, drizzled with fat-free lemon yogurt.

Vegetable oil spray

Topping

1½ cups fresh or frozen blueberries (small wild blueberries preferred)

¼ cup firmly packed light brown sugar

¼ teaspoon ground cinnamon

Cake

2 cups all-purpose flour

1 cup whole-wheat pastry flour

1 teaspoon baking powder

½ teaspoon baking soda

¼ teaspoon ground cardamom

¼ teaspoon ground nutmeg

1 cup sugar

1 cup fat-free or low-fat plain yogurt (8 ounces)

Egg substitute equivalent to 3 eggs, or 3 large eggs

¼ cup fat-free milk

3 tablespoons acceptable vegetable oil

¼ cup plus 1 tablespoon unsweetened applesauce

1½ teaspoons grated lemon zest

½ teaspoon vanilla extract

Set oven temperature to 350° F. Spray a 13 x 9 x 2-inch baking pan with vegetable oil spray; set aside.

In a small bowl, combine topping ingredients.

For cake, in a medium bowl, combine all-purpose flour, pastry flour, baking powder, baking soda, cardamom, and nutmeg.

In a large bowl, whisk together remaining ingredients. Add flour mixture, stirring until flour is moistened. Pour batter into baking pan. Sprinkle with topping.

Bake for 30 minutes, or until a toothpick inserted near center comes out clean. Cool on a cooling rack for 10 to 20 minutes before slicing.

Raspberry Coffeecake

Substitute 1 cup fresh raspberries for blueberries and ½ teaspoon almond extract for lemon zest and vanilla extract. (Calories 188; Protein 5 g; Carbohydrates 36 g; Cholesterol 0 mg; Total Fat 3 g; Saturated 0 g; Polyunsaturated —; Monounsaturated —; Fiber 2 g; Sodium 93 mg)

Cook's Tip on Whole-Wheat Pastry Flour

Whole-wheat pastry flour contains less gluten than regular whole-wheat flour. Therefore, it's lighter and better in cakes and pastries. It is available in health food and gourmet markets and in some supermarkets.

(PER SERVING)

Calories 192

Protein 5 g

Carbohydrates 37 g

Cholesterol 0 mg

Total Fat 3 g

Saturated 0 g

Polyunsaturated —

Monounsaturated —

Fiber 2 g

Sodium 94 mg

Mini Cinnamon Stackups

- Serves 4; 1 waffle and ½ cup yogurt per serving
- Preparation time: 5 minutes
- Cooking time: 5 minutes

Have fun at breakfast with this terrific taste combination of mini waffles, cinnamon-sugared fruits, and yogurt. Or serve later in the day with frozen yogurt as a different way to enjoy an old-fashioned ice cream "cone."

4 4-piece frozen mini waffles

1 tablespoon sugar

¼ teaspoon ground cinnamon

2 kiwifruit

1 star fruit (optional)

2 cups fat-free or low-fat vanilla yogurt, frozen vanilla yogurt, or vanilla ice cream

½ cup fresh blueberries

1 cup fresh raspberries or strawberries

Toast waffles and separate each into four pieces. Arrange three pieces in a cloverleaf on each of four plates.

Meanwhile, in a small bowl, combine sugar and cinnamon. Cut each kiwifruit crosswise into six pieces. Cut star fruit crosswise into eight pieces.

To assemble, sprinkle half the cinnamon sugar over waffles. Spoon ½ cup yogurt onto each serving. Arrange three slices kiwifruit, two slices star fruit, 2 tablespoons blueberries, and ¼ cup raspberries on each. Angle remaining waffles on side of fruit and sprinkle with remaining cinnamon sugar.

(PER SERVING)

Calories 227

Protein 8 g

Carbohydrates 43 g

Cholesterol 10 mg

Total Fat 3 g

Saturated 1 g

Polyunsaturated —

Monounsaturated —

Fiber 5 g

Sodium 266 mg

Yogurt Brûlée with Blueberries

Serves 4; 1 cup per serving ∎
Preparation time: 5 minutes ∎
Cooking time: 2 to 4 minutes ∎

This breakfast treat looks so elegant, your family will think it took hours instead of minutes to prepare. You can also serve this as dessert, but caution is advised: You may be tempted to eat dessert first!

2 cups fresh or 4 cups unsweetened
  frozen blueberries, thawed

1 teaspoon grated lemon zest

2 8-ounce containers fat-free or
  low-fat vanilla yogurt (2 cups)

2 tablespoons plus 2 teaspoons brown
  sugar

Preheat broiler. Put four 1-cup custard cups or ramekins on a broilerproof baking sheet.

In a medium bowl, stir together blueberries and lemon zest.

To assemble, spoon ½ cup blueberry mixture into each custard cup. Top each with about ½ cup yogurt and 2 teaspoons brown sugar.

Broil about 4 inches from heat for 2 to 4 minutes, or until brown sugar is melted and bubbly. Watch carefully to keep sugar from burning.

Cook's Tip

One way to thaw frozen blueberries is in the microwave. Measure them into a microwave-safe container. Microwave on 50 percent (medium) power for 4 to 5 minutes (no stirring needed). This method preserves the juice, which you can spoon in with the berries.

(PER SERVING)

Calories 143

Protein 5 g

Carbohydrates 31 g

Cholesterol 2 mg

Total Fat 0 g

  Saturated 0 g

  Polyunsaturated 0 g

  Monounsaturated 0 g

Fiber 2 g

Sodium 69 mg

Fruitful Brown Rice Cereal

- Serves 4; ⅔ cup per serving
- Preparation time: 5 minutes
- Cooking time: 15 minutes

This sweet, fragrant breakfast dish is so full of flavor that your kids won't know it's good for them. Topped with slices of banana or strawberries and additional milk, it's even more delicious and healthful.

Vegetable oil spray

1¼ cups low-fat vanilla soy milk or 1¼ cups fat-free milk and 1 teaspoon vanilla extract

1 cup unsweetened apple juice

2 cups instant brown rice

¼ cup dried fruit, such as currants, cherries, blueberries, or raisins, or a combination

1 teaspoon ground cinnamon

Spray a medium saucepan with vegetable oil spray. Pour milk and apple juice into pan; bring to a boil over high heat, about 4 minutes.

Stir remaining ingredients into pan. Reduce heat and simmer, covered, for 10 minutes, or until liquids are absorbed and rice is tender.

(PER SERVING)

Calories 246

Protein 6 g

Carbohydrates 53 g

Cholesterol 0 mg

Total Fat 2 g

  Saturated 0 g

  Polyunsaturated —

  Monounsaturated —

Fiber 2 g

Sodium 53 mg

Huevos Rancheros Casserole

Serves 6; ¾ cup per serving ■
Preparation time: 15 minutes ■
Cooking time: 49 to 50 minutes ■

Capture the traditional flavors of huevos rancheros with this any-time-of-day casserole. You can make it and bake it right away, or prepare it ahead of time and bake it the next day.

Vegetable oil spray

2 ounces turkey breakfast sausage, casings removed (2 links)

1 Anaheim pepper, seeded and diced

6 6-inch corn tortillas, diced

15-ounce can no-salt-added black beans, rinsed and drained

1 cup cherry tomatoes, halved

2 cups fat-free milk

Egg substitute equivalent to 6 eggs

2 tablespoons sliced black olives, drained

Preheat oven to 350° F. Lightly spray a 9-inch square baking pan with vegetable oil spray; set aside.

In a small nonstick skillet, cook sausage over medium-high heat for 3 minutes, stirring to break up. Add pepper and cook for 1 to 2 minutes, or until pepper is tender and sausage is no longer pink. Put in a colander and rinse with hot water; drain well. Put in baking pan.

Top with tortillas, then with beans, and finally with tomatoes.

In a medium bowl, whisk together milk and egg substitute. Pour over casserole.

Bake for 45 minutes, or until center is set. Cut into six pieces and sprinkle with olives.

COOK'S TIP

To make the casserole ahead of time, assemble as directed, then cover and refrigerate for up to 12 hours before baking. Remove from refrigerator 15 minutes before baking.

(PER SERVING)

Calories 207

Protein 16 g

Carbohydrates 31 g

Cholesterol 7 mg

Total Fat 2 g

   Saturated 1 g

   Polyunsaturated 1 g

   Monounsaturated 0 g

Fiber 5 g

Sodium 250 mg

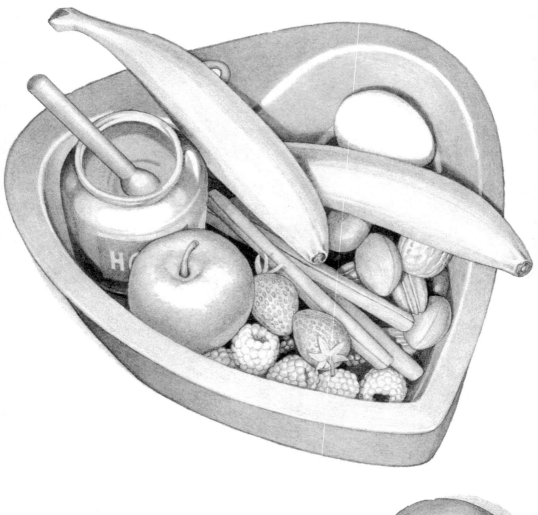
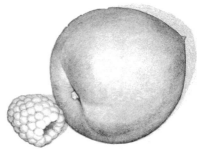

DESSERTS

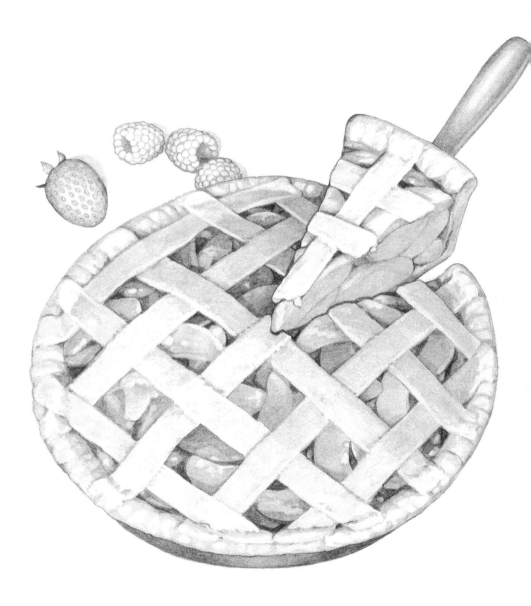

Chocolate Pudding Cake

Chocolate Hazelnut Angel Food
Cake with Bananas

    Chocolate Walnut Angel Food
    Cake with Raspberries

    Chocolate Almond Angel
    Food Cake with Oranges

    Chocolate Pistachio Angel
    Food Cake with Strawberries

Devil's Food Cake
with Caramel Drizzles

    Spice Cake with Caramel
    Drizzles

Lemon Cake with Apricot Glaze

    Lemon Cake with Apricot
    Topping

    Lemon Cupcakes with Apricot
    Glaze

Nectarine and Raspberry Pie
with Phyllo Crust

Heavenly Frozen Angel Food
and Berry Pie

Pear Crisp

Ginger Snacks

    Ginger Banana Snacks

Cinnamon Apple Bars

Bread Pudding with Peaches
and Bourbon Sauce

Ambrosia Parfait

Cranberry Cinnamon Baked
Apples

Two-Way Strawberry Freeze

    Two-Way Mixed-Fruit Freeze

Frozen Dessert Terrine

Mango and Raspberry Fruit
Sauces

Cheesecake Sauce

Apricot Dessert Sauce

Chocolate Pudding Cake

Serves 24; 1 square per serving ■
Preparation time: 20 minutes ■
Baking time: 35 to 40 minutes ■
Standing time: 15 minutes ■

You'll be surprised at the rich pool of fudge sauce that works its way to the bottom of this cake as it bakes. This decadent dessert is best when served warm, but you won't be able to resist it even at room temperature.

Vegetable oil spray

Cake

2 cups all-purpose flour

1½ cups sugar

½ cup unsweetened cocoa powder

1 tablespoon plus 1 teaspoon baking powder

¼ teaspoon salt

1 cup fat-free milk

½ cup unsweetened applesauce

2 teaspoons vanilla extract

Pudding

2 cups boiling water

1½ cups firmly packed light brown sugar

½ cup unsweetened cocoa powder

Preheat oven to 350° F. Spray a 13 x 9 x 2-inch baking pan with vegetable oil spray; set aside.

In a large bowl, whisk together flour, sugar, cocoa, baking powder, and salt. Whisk in remaining cake ingredients, blending thoroughly. Pour into baking pan, spreading evenly.

In a large bowl, whisk together pudding ingredients until sugar and cocoa are dissolved. Pour carefully over batter. (Pudding layer will be thin and runny.)

Bake for 35 to 40 minutes, or until top is firm to the touch. (A toothpick inserted in center of cake won't be an accurate test for doneness.) Let cake rest for 15 minutes before cutting. To serve, slice cake and top with sauce, or pool sauce on plate and top with cake. Cover and refrigerate leftovers for up to 7 days or wrap tightly and freeze for up to 2 months.

(PER SERVING)

Calories 152

Protein 2 g

Carbohydrates 37 g

Cholesterol 0 mg

Total Fat 1 g

  Saturated 0 g

   Polyunsaturated 0 g

   Monounsaturated 0 g

Fiber 2 g

Sodium 94 mg

Chocolate Hazelnut Angel Food Cake with Bananas

- Serves 16; 2 slices per serving
- Preparation time: 10 minutes
- Cooking time: 33 to 43 minutes
- Cooling time: 30 minutes

With this recipe, you'll get a bonus—twice. First, you get a chocolate layer in addition to a traditional layer of angel food cake. Second, you get two cakes, enough so you can enjoy one now and freeze one for later.

16-ounce package angel food cake mix

2 tablespoons cocoa powder (dark, European-style preferred)

¾ cup water (or half the amount called for in package directions)

2 teaspoons hazelnut syrup

¾ cup water (or half the amount called for in package directions)

1 cup fat-free hot fudge topping

1 tablespoon hazelnut syrup

8 medium bananas

⅓ cup chopped hazelnuts

(PER SERVING)

Calories 231

Protein 4 g

Carbohydrates 51 g

Cholesterol 0 mg

Total Fat 2 g

  Saturated 0 g

  Polyunsaturated 0 g

  Monounsaturated 1 g

Fiber 1 g

Sodium 239 mg

Preheat oven to 350° F (or use package directions).

Divide cake mix in half; put each half in a separate medium mixing bowl (using a scale or measuring cup is recommended).

For chocolate layer, stir cocoa powder into half the cake mix.

In a small bowl, combine ¾ cup water and 2 teaspoons syrup; pour into chocolate mixture. Beat with an electric mixer on low speed until liquid is absorbed, about 30 seconds. Increase speed to medium and beat for exactly 1 minute (or use package directions).

Divide chocolate mixture evenly between two 9 x 5-inch loaf pans (don't spray with vegetable oil spray).

For white layer, pour ¾ cup water into remaining cake mix. Beat with an electric mixer on low speed until liquid is absorbed, about 30 seconds. Increase speed to medium and beat for exactly 1 minute (or use package directions). Gently pour onto chocolate layers. Using a knife, cut through both layers in a crisscross pattern to create a slightly swirled effect.

Bake for 33 to 43 minutes (or use package directions), or until a toothpick inserted in center comes out clean.

Place loaf pans on their sides on a cooling rack and let sit for 30 minutes, or until cooled. Run a spatula around sides of pan to loosen cakes. Invert cakes on a cutting board and cut each cake into 16 slices. (Cake can be frozen, whole or sliced, for up to 4 months.)

In a small saucepan, heat fudge topping and 1 tablespoon syrup over low heat for 1 to 2 minutes, or until warmed through, stirring occasionally.

Slice bananas.

To serve, place 2 pieces of cake on a dessert plate and top with ½ cup banana slices. Drizzle 1 tablespoon hot fudge mixture over bananas and sprinkle with nuts. Repeat with remaining ingredients.

CHOCOLATE WALNUT ANGEL FOOD CAKE WITH RASPBERRIES

For the listed syrup, fruit, and nuts, substitute 1 tablespoon plus 2 teaspoons raspberry syrup (divided use); 8 cups raspberries (about 4½ pints); and ⅓ cup chopped walnuts (about 1½ ounces). (Calories 209; Protein 5 g; Carbohydrates 45 g; Cholesterol 0 mg; Total Fat 2 g; Saturated 0 g; Polyunsaturated 1 g; Monounsaturated 0 g; Fiber 5 g; Sodium 239 mg)

CHOCOLATE ALMOND ANGEL FOOD CAKE WITH ORANGES

For the listed syrup, fruit, and nuts, substitute 1 tablespoon plus 2 teaspoons orange syrup (divided use); 8 cups mandarin oranges, canned in water or light syrup, drained; and ⅓ cup sliced almonds (about 1 ounce). (Calories 224; Protein 5 g; Carbohydrates 49 g; Cholesterol 0 mg; Total Fat 2 g; Saturated 0 g; Polyunsaturated 0 g; Monounsaturated 1 g; Fiber 3 g; Sodium 240 mg)

CHOCOLATE PISTACHIO ANGEL FOOD CAKE WITH STRAWBERRIES

For the listed syrup, fruit, and nuts, substitute 1 table-spoon plus 2 teaspoons chocolate syrup (divided use); 8 cups sliced strawberries (about 1 quart whole berries); and ⅓ cup pistachios. (Calories 219; Protein 5 g; Carbohydrates 48 g; Cholesterol 0 mg; Total Fat 2 g; Saturated 0 g; Polyunsaturated 1 g; Monounsaturated 1 g; Fiber 4 g; Sodium 241 mg)

COOK'S TIP ON FLAVORED SYRUPS

Flavored syrups, primarily used to flavor coffee (and usually found in the coffee aisle of grocery or specialty stores), can also add fat-free flavor to your favorite pies, cakes, and cookies, as well as to whipped topping. Use small amounts (teaspoons) at first; then adjust to taste.

Devil's Food Cake with Caramel Drizzles

Serves 20; 1 slice per serving ■
Preparation time: 5 minutes ■
Cooking time: 28 minutes ■

Ultramoist and ultratender, this chocolate cake disappears quickly.

Vegetable oil spray

18.25-ounce box light devil's food
   cake mix

Whites of 6 large eggs, egg substitute
   equivalent to 3 eggs, or 3 large eggs

2 4-ounce jars baby food pureed
   prunes

1 cup cold coffee or water

½ cup fat-free caramel topping or
   sifted confectioners' sugar

Preheat oven to 350° F. Spray a 15 x 11-inch jelly-roll pan with vegetable oil spray.

In a large bowl, combine all ingredients except caramel topping, using package directions (prunes replace oil). Pour batter into pan and spread evenly.

Bake using package directions. Place pan on cooling rack and let cool slightly.

Just before serving, drizzle each piece with 1 teaspoon caramel topping or dust with confectioners' sugar. Serve warm or at room temperature.

SPICE CAKE WITH CARAMEL DRIZZLES

Substitute spice cake mix for devil's food cake mix, pureed carrots for prunes, and unsweetened apple juice or orange juice for coffee. (Calories 135; Protein 2 g; Carbohydrates 31 g; Cholesterol 0 mg; Total Fat 1 g; Saturated 0 g; Polyunsaturated 0 g; Monounsaturated 0 g; Fiber 0 g; Sodium 211 mg)

(PER SERVING)

Calories 134

Protein 2 g

Carbohydrates 30 g

Cholesterol 0 mg

Total Fat 1 g

  Saturated 0 g

  Polyunsaturated 0 g

  Monounsaturated 0 g

Fiber 1 g

Sodium 262 mg

Lemon Cake with Apricot Glaze

- Serves 16; 1 slice per serving
- Preparation time: 20 minutes
- Cooking time: 17 minutes

Lemon juice and zest give this cake a refreshing taste. The sweetness of the apricot preserves balances the tartness of the lemon.

Vegetable oil spray

18.25-ounce package lemon-flavored cake mix

Whites of 6 large eggs, egg substitute equivalent to 3 eggs, or 3 large eggs

½ cup water

1 tablespoon plus 1½ teaspoons lemon zest

¼ cup plus 2 tablespoons lemon juice (2 medium lemons)

¾ cup all-fruit apricot preserves

1 cup frozen fat-free or light whipped topping, thawed

Preheat oven to 325° F. Spray a 13 x 9 x 2-inch baking pan with vegetable oil spray.

In a large mixing bowl, combine cake mix, egg whites, water, zest, and lemon juice. Mix using package directions. Pour batter into pan.

Bake for 25 to 30 minutes, or until toothpick inserted in center comes out clean. Put on cooling rack.

In a small saucepan, heat preserves over medium-high heat until melted, 1 to 2 minutes, stirring constantly. Brush evenly over cake.

Serve warm or at room temperature with 1 tablespoon whipped topping on each piece.

LEMON CAKE WITH APRICOT TOPPING

Beat unheated preserves with a fork, if desired. Fold into 3 cups frozen fat-free or light whipped topping, thawed; spread over completely cooled cake. Refrigerate leftovers. (Calories 191; Protein 2 g; Carbohydrates 39 g; Cholesterol 0 mg; Total Fat 3 g; Saturated 1 g; Polyunsaturated 0 g; Monounsaturated 2 g; Fiber 0 g; Sodium 211 mg)

Lemon Cupcakes with Apricot Glaze

For cupcakes, pour batter into two 12-cup muffin pans. Follow baking times on package. Brush with glaze. Increase amount of whipped topping to 1½ cups. (Calories 122; Protein 1 g; Carbohydrates 25 g; Cholesterol 0 mg; Total Fat 2 g; Saturated 1 g; Polyunsaturated 0 g; Monounsaturated 1 g; Fiber 0 g; Sodium 139 mg)

Cook's Tip on Citrus Zest

An implement called a zester makes quick work of removing the peel, or zest, of citrus fruit. Use rather firm downward strokes, being careful not to get any of the pith, the bitter white layer just beneath the peel. Measuring and cleanup will be easy if you work over a sheet of wax paper.

(PER SERVING)
Calories 179
Protein 2 g
Carbohydrates 36 g
Cholesterol 0 mg
Total Fat 3 g
  Saturated 1 g
  Polyunsaturated 0 g
  Monounsaturated 2 g
Fiber 0 g
Sodium 206 mg

Nectarine and Raspberry Pie with Phyllo Crust

- Serves 8; 1 slice per serving
- Preparation time: 20 minutes
- Cooking time: 30 minutes

Celebrate summer with this fresh-fruit pie. Or if you have the winter blues, use frozen peaches and raspberries to perk up your spirits and remind yourself that spring will soon arrive.

Filling

6 medium nectarines, sliced (about 2 pounds), or 4 cups frozen sliced peaches, thawed

1¼ cups fresh or frozen raspberries, thawed (about ¾ pint fresh or 12 ounces frozen)

¼ cup honey

2 tablespoons light margarine, softened

1 teaspoon grated lemon zest

1 tablespoon lemon juice

¼ teaspoon ground nutmeg

Crust

2 tablespoons sugar

½ teaspoon ground cinnamon

Butter-flavor vegetable oil spray

6 sheets frozen phyllo dough, thawed

In a large bowl, stir together filling ingredients; set aside.

For crust, stir together sugar and cinnamon in a small bowl; set aside.

Preheat oven to 375° F. Spray a 9-inch pie plate with vegetable oil spray.

Stack phyllo sheets on a cutting board. Cut sheets all at once into a 12-inch square, keeping leftover strips. Place 1 sheet of phyllo in pie plate. Lightly spray with vegetable oil spray. Sprinkle with 1 teaspoon sugar mixture. Repeat with remaining ingredients. Either layer leftover strips over phyllo sheets or save for making a lattice crust.

Spoon filling into crust. Crisscross strips for a lattice crust, if desired.

Bake for 30 minutes, or until fruit is tender and phyllo is golden brown.

COOK'S TIP ON PHYLLO

Phyllo (FEE-loh), available frozen in most large supermarkets and specialty groceries, is a tissue-thin pastry dough. To thaw, put frozen phyllo dough in the refrigerator for about 6 hours. Thawed phyllo sheets quickly become dry and brittle, so use a damp dish towel to cover the dough you aren't using. Unopened thawed dough will keep in the refrigerator for about a month. If refrozen, phyllo dough can become brittle and crumbly.

(PER SERVING)

Calories 149

Protein 2 g

Carbohydrates 34 g

Cholesterol 0 mg

Total Fat 2 g

　Saturated 0 g

　Polyunsaturated 1 g

　Monounsaturated 0 g

Fiber 3 g

Sodium 71 mg

Heavenly Frozen Angel Food and Berry Pie

- Serves 10; 1 slice per serving
- Preparation time: 20 minutes
- Freezing time: 3 hours
- Thawing time: 20 to 25 minutes

This heavenly pie combines chocolate and berries for a frozen taste treat.

Vegetable oil spray

1 pound 2 ounces angel food cake, cubed (about 12 cups)

½ cup chocolate-flavored sweetened condensed milk

½ cup fat-free sweetened condensed milk

2 cups frozen sweetened raspberries (20 ounces)

1 cup frozen unsweetened blackberries (8 ounces)

1 cup frozen fat-free or light whipped topping, thawed

2 tablespoons grenadine

Spray a 9-inch pie plate with vegetable oil spray; set aside.

Put cake in a medium bowl. Pour condensed milks over cake. Stir or use your hands to mix milks into cake. (Cake will condense in size and turn a chocolate color when properly mixed. If a few white streaks of cake remain, that's acceptable.)

In a medium bowl, stir together raspberries and blackberries.

In a small bowl, stir together whipped topping and grenadine.

To assemble, press half the cake mixture into pie plate. Top with half the berries. Repeat layers. Spread topping mixture over berries. Stick five toothpicks into pie (one in center, four around edge), then cover with plastic wrap (let it rest on toothpicks).

Freeze pie for 3 hours, or until firm.

To serve, cut frozen pie with a sharp knife. (To make cutting easier, run knife under hot water and dry before slicing.) Let soften for 20 to 25 minutes before serving.

(PER SERVING)

Calories 309

Protein 6 g

Carbohydrates 69 g

Cholesterol 5 mg

Total Fat 1 g

  Saturated 1 g

  Polyunsaturated 0 g

  Monounsaturated 0 g

Fiber 4 g

Sodium 194 mg

Pear Crisp

Serves 6; ½ cup per serving ■
Preparation time: 15 minutes ■
Cooking time: 28 minutes ■
Cooling time: 20 minutes ■

Keep a big can of pears in the pantry, and you can enjoy this simple, spicy crisp any time.

29-ounce can pears or sliced peaches in fruit juice

¼ cup dry white wine (regular or nonalcoholic), pear juice, or peach juice

2 tablespoons sugar

¼ teaspoon ground ginger

¼ teaspoon ground cloves or ground cinnamon

Topping

¼ cup chopped pecans (about 1 ounce)

½ cup uncooked rolled oats

½ cup firmly packed light brown sugar

2 tablespoons whole-wheat pastry flour or all-purpose flour

¼ teaspoon ground nutmeg

2 teaspoons acceptable vegetable oil

Preheat oven to 350° F.

Drain pears, reserving ½ cup juice. Slice pears and put in a 1-quart casserole dish or 9-inch pie plate.

In a medium saucepan, stir together juice, wine, sugar, ginger, and cloves; bring to a boil over medium-high heat. Cook for 4 minutes, or until reduced by half, stirring occasionally.

Meanwhile, dry-roast pecans in preheating oven for about 10 minutes, or until golden brown.

In a small bowl, mix remaining topping ingredients except oil. Using a fork, stir in oil, then pecans. Sprinkle topping over pears. Pour sauce over all.

Bake for 20 minutes, or until top is lightly browned and sauce is bubbly. Cool for 20 minutes before serving.

VARIATION

For apple crisp, use canned apple slices, replace ginger with ⅛ teaspoon nutmeg, and use cinnamon, not cloves.

(PER SERVING)

Calories 216

Protein 2 g

Carbohydrates 41 g

Cholesterol 0 mg

Total Fat 5 g

    Saturated 1 g

    Polyunsaturated 2 g

    Monounsaturated 2 g

Fiber 4 g

Sodium 10 mg

Ginger Snacks

- Serves 16; 1 muffin per serving
- Preparation time: 15 minutes
- Cooking time: 25 minutes

Baked with pumpkin for added flavor, moisture, and body, these gingerbread muffins are perfect for brown-bag or after-school snacks.

Vegetable oil spray

14.5- or 15-ounce box gingerbread mix

1¼ cups orange juice (4 medium oranges) or water

Whites of 2 large eggs, egg substitute equivalent to 1 egg, or 1 large egg

1 cup canned pumpkin

¾ teaspoon ground cinnamon

1 tablespoon plus 1½ teaspoons sugar

¼ teaspoon ground cinnamon

Preheat oven to 350° F. Spray 16 nonstick muffin cups with vegetable oil spray. (Pour several tablespoons of water into unused cups to keep pan from warping.)

Put cake mix, orange juice, and egg whites in a large mixing bowl. Mix using package directions.

Stir in pumpkin and ¾ teaspoon cinnamon. Spoon batter into muffin cups.

Bake for 25 minutes, or until muffin springs back slightly when you press slightly on center.

Meanwhile, combine sugar with cinnamon.

When muffins are done, put pan on cooling rack and sprinkle muffins with sugar mixture.

(PER SERVING)

Calories 132

Protein 2 g

Carbohydrates 24 g

Cholesterol 0 mg

Total Fat 3 g

  Saturated 1 g

  Polyunsaturated 0 g

  Monounsaturated 1 g

Fiber 1 g

Sodium 179 mg

GINGER BANANA SNACKS

Substitute 1 cup mashed ripe banana for pumpkin, apple juice for orange juice, and nutmeg for cinnamon. (Calories 140; Protein 2 g; Carbohydrates 26 g; Cholesterol 0 mg; Total Fat 3 g; Saturated 1 g; Polyunsaturated 0 g; Monounsaturated 1 g; Fiber 0 g; Sodium 179 mg)

Cinnamon Apple Bars

Serves 18; 2 per serving ■
Preparation time: 15 minutes ■
Cooking time: 20 minutes ■
Cooling time: 10 minutes ■

The exquisite aroma of cinnamon, apples, and brown sugar baking will make it hard to wait for this treat to come out of the oven.

Vegetable oil spray

2 cups all-purpose flour

1½ teaspoons baking powder

1 teaspoon ground cinnamon

¼ teaspoon baking soda

1 cup drained canned unsweetened apple slices or drained canned pears in fruit juice, cut into ½-inch pieces

¾ cup firmly packed light brown sugar

½ cup cranberry applesauce or unsweetened applesauce

Egg substitute equivalent to 2 eggs, or 2 large eggs

¼ cup sugar

2 tablespoons acceptable vegetable oil

1 teaspoon vanilla extract

Preheat oven to 350° F. Spray a 13 x 9 x 2-inch baking pan with vegetable oil spray.

In a medium bowl, stir together flour, baking powder, cinnamon, and baking soda.

In another medium bowl, stir together remaining ingredients. Add flour mixture, stirring until just moistened. Pour batter into baking pan.

Bake for 20 minutes, or until a knife inserted in the center comes out clean. Let cool on cooling rack for 10 minutes, then cut into 36 bars.

(PER SERVING)

Calories 123

Protein 2 g

Carbohydrates 25 g

Cholesterol 0 mg

Total Fat 2 g

   Saturated 0 g

   Polyunsaturated 1 g

   Monounsaturated 0 g

Fiber 1 g

Sodium 59 mg

Bread Pudding with Peaches and Bourbon Sauce

- Serves 8; ½ cup pudding and ¼ cup sauce per serving
- Preparation time: 15 minutes
- Cooking time: 30 to 35 minutes

Grace your dinner table with this show-stopping dessert. It's the perfect end to a southern meal.

Butter-flavor vegetable oil spray

Pudding

2 tablespoons fat-free margarine

8 ½-inch slices baguette-style French bread (about 3 ounces)

½ teaspoon ground cinnamon

2 cups unsweetened sliced frozen peaches, thawed (20 ounces), or peeled, sliced fresh peaches (about 3 medium)

2 tablespoons dried cherries, raisins, or dried blueberries (optional)

Egg substitute equivalent to 2 eggs, or 2 large eggs

1 cup fat-free milk

¼ to ½ cup sugar

Bourbon Sauce

½ small package (about 3.1 ounces) fat-free, sugar-free vanilla cook and serve pudding mix (about 4 tablespoons plus 1½ teaspoons)

1 cup fat-free milk

1 tablespoon bourbon or rum, or ¼ teaspoon rum flavoring

Preheat oven to 350° F. Lightly spray eight 6-ounce glass or porcelain custard cups or a 9-inch square non-stick baking pan with vegetable oil spray. If using custard cups, put on a baking sheet.

For pudding, spread a thin layer of margarine on one side of each bread slice; put spread side up on a cutting board.

Sprinkle bread with cinnamon. Cut into ½-inch cubes and put in custard cups.

Spoon ¼ cup peaches into each cup; sprinkle with cherries.

In a medium bowl, whisk together egg substitute, 1 cup milk, and ¼ to ½ cup sugar (depending on sweetness of peaches). Pour into custard cups.

Bake for 30 to 35 minutes, or until center of pudding is set. (If using custard cups, leave them on baking sheet.)

About 10 minutes before pudding is done, prepare sauce. In a medium saucepan, whisk together pudding mix and milk until well blended, 30 to 60 seconds. Bring to a boil over medium-high heat, 2 to 3 minutes, whisking occasionally.

Reduce heat to medium-low and whisk in bourbon; cook for 1 to 2 minutes, until thickened. Keep sauce warm over low heat until pudding is done. (Sauce thickens more as it cools.)

To serve, spoon about ¼ cup sauce over each pudding. Or spoon sauce onto dessert plates, slide a spatula around sides of custard cups, remove puddings with a spoon, and place on sauce.

(PER SERVING)

Calories 155

Protein 5 g

Carbohydrates 26 g

Cholesterol 1 mg

Total Fat 0 g

Saturated 0 g

Polyunsaturated 0 g

Monounsaturated 0 g

Fiber 1 g

Sodium 176 mg

Ambrosia Parfait

- Serves 6; 1 cup per serving
- Preparation time: 15 minutes

Here's a modern twist to a comforting favorite. It's perfect not only for dessert but also as a starter for a summer brunch.

1 cup cubed fresh or bottled mango

1 medium banana, sliced

11-ounce can mandarin oranges in water or light syrup, drained

8-ounce can pineapple tidbits in their own juice, drained

½ cup sliced strawberries

1 tablespoon shredded coconut

3 8-ounce containers fat-free or low-fat lemon yogurt (3 cups)

2 tablespoons dried cranberries (optional)

In a medium bowl, combine mango, banana, mandarin oranges, pineapple, strawberries, and coconut.

To assemble, spoon about ¼ cup yogurt into each of six parfait glasses or small bowls. Top each with ¼ cup fruit mixture. Repeat. Sprinkle with cranberries. Parfaits can be covered and refrigerated for up to 4 hours before serving.

(PER SERVING)

Calories 167

Protein 6 g

Carbohydrates 34 g

Cholesterol 2 mg

Total Fat 1 g

  Saturated 0 g

  Polyunsaturated 0 g

  Monounsaturated 0 g

Fiber 3 g

Sodium 67 mg

Cranberry Cinnamon Baked Apples

Serves 4; 1/2 apple per serving ■
Preparation time: 10 minutes ■
Cooking time: 35 to 40 minutes ■

As the apples bake, their juice combines with brown sugar and orange juice to create a light caramel sauce.

Vegetable oil spray

2 8-ounce baking apples, such as Rome Beauty, Winesap, or Stayman, halved and cored

½ cup dried cranberries

3 tablespoons orange juice, unsweetened apple juice, or water

2 tablespoons chopped pecans

2 tablespoons dark brown sugar

1 teaspoon vanilla, butter, and nut flavoring or vanilla extract

1 teaspoon ground cinnamon

Preheat oven to 350° F. Spray an 8-inch square nonstick baking pan with vegetable oil spray.

Put halved apples in pan. (If needed to keep apples from rocking, cut a very thin slice off bottom of each half.)

In a small bowl, stir together remaining ingredients. Spoon onto each apple half. Cover pan with aluminum foil.

Bake for 10 minutes; remove foil and bake for 25 to 30 minutes, or until apples are easily pierced with a fork.

(PER SERVING)

Calories 149

Protein 1 g

Carbohydrates 33 g

Cholesterol 0 mg

Total Fat 3 g

   Saturated 0 g

   Polyunsaturated 1 g

   Monounsaturated 1 g

Fiber 3 g

Sodium 2 mg

Two-Way Strawberry Freeze

- Serves 11; ½ cup per serving
- Preparation time: 5 minutes
- Freezing time (optional): 1 hour

Blend sweet strawberries with white grape juice and a bit of wine for a fruity drink or a refreshing ice.

2 cups white grape juice

16 ounces frozen unsweetened strawberries (about 3 cups)

1 cup dry white wine (regular or nonalcoholic) or ginger ale (regular or diet)

In a blender or food processor, blend grape juice and strawberries until smooth.

Slowly add wine, blending until smooth.

Serve immediately as a beverage or seal in a large airtight plastic bag and lay bag flat in freezer until semisoft, about 1 hour.

TWO-WAY MIXED-FRUIT FREEZE

Substitute 2 cups pineapple-orange juice for grape juice; 1 pound frozen mixed melon or mixed fruit for strawberries; and 1 cup lemon-lime soda or 1 tablespoon sugar and ¼ cup lemon juice for wine. Blend as directed above. Serve immediately or freeze until semisoft. (Calories 47; Protein 1 g; Carbohydrates 11 g; Cholesterol 0 mg; Total Fat 0 g; Saturated 0 g; Polyunsaturated 0 g; Monounsaturated 0 g; Fiber 0 g; Sodium 19 mg)

COOK'S TIP ON FREEZING LIQUIDS

Laying a bag of liquid flat in the freezer helps the liquid freeze faster.

(PER SERVING)

Calories 57

Protein 0 g

Carbohydrates 11 g

Cholesterol 0 mg

Total Fat 0 g

Saturated 0 g

Polyunsaturated 0 g

Monounsaturated 0 g

Fiber 1 g

Sodium 3 mg

Frozen Dessert Terrine

Serves 10; 1 slice per serving ■
Preparation time: 20 minutes ■
Freezing time: 3 hours to 1 week ■

Perfect for a dinner party, this tricolor terrine can be made up to a week in advance. Experiment with different sherbets, sorbets, and frozen yogurts for new flavor and color combinations.

1½ cups fat-free chocolate sorbet

1½ cups orange sherbet

2½ cups fat-free frozen vanilla yogurt (20 ounces)

¼ cup chocolate syrup

Let sorbet, sherbet, and frozen yogurt soften for 4 to 5 minutes. Meanwhile, line an 8½ x 4½ x 2½-inch loaf pan with plastic wrap.

Using a spatula, spread sorbet evenly in loaf pan. Spread sherbet over chocolate layer. Spread yogurt over orange layer. Cover with plastic wrap and freeze for 3 hours to 1 week.

To serve, drizzle about 1 teaspoon chocolate syrup over each dessert plate. Remove plastic wrap cover from terrine and invert onto a cutting board. Remove remaining plastic wrap. Cut terrine into 10 slices. Place on prepared plates.

(PER SERVING)

Calories 149

Protein 2 g

Carbohydrates 34 g

Cholesterol 2 mg

Total Fat 1 g

  Saturated 0 g

  Polyunsaturated 0 g

  Monounsaturated 0 g

Fiber 1 g

Sodium 64 mg

Mango and Raspberry Fruit Sauces

- Serves 16; 2 tablespoons plus 1½ teaspoons per serving
- Preparation time: 20 minutes

Let the creativity flow when you use these contrasting sauces. To add an elegant touch to angel food cake or reduced-fat pound cake, use a cookie cutter to cut shapes from slices of the cake; then place the cake on the sauces. You can also top the sauces with poached pears or sliced fresh fruit or use them as a topping for fat-free frozen yogurt, sherbet, or sorbet or even on pancakes or French toast.

12 ounces frozen raspberries (about 1¼ cups)

26-ounce jar refrigerated mango slices or 3 medium mangoes

2 tablespoons canned strawberry-banana nectar, or to taste

1 tablespoon honey

2 tablespoons canned peach nectar, or to taste

Place unopened bag of frozen raspberries in a bowl of cold water. Let sit at room temperature, turning occasionally, for about 10 minutes.

Meanwhile, drain mango slices or slice mangoes.

Put raspberries with their liquid, strawberry-banana nectar, and honey in a food processor or blender. Process for about 30 seconds, or until smooth (except seeds). Pour into a fine-mesh strainer; using a rubber scraper, push through into a bowl. Transfer mixture to a syrup dispenser or plastic squeeze bottle. Discard seeds. Cover and refrigerate mixture until ready to use.

Thoroughly rinse work bowl and blade of food processor or blender. Process mango slices and peach nectar for about 30 seconds, or until smooth. Pour into a bowl, syrup dispenser, or squeeze bottle.

To serve, spoon about 1 tablespoon plus 1½ teaspoons mango sauce onto a dessert plate. Tilt plate slightly to spread mixture evenly. Spoon about 1 tablespoon raspberry sauce beside mango sauce or drizzle it over mango sauce in a decorative pattern (a squeeze bottle lets you "paint" a striking contrasting design).

Cook's Tip

The nectars are used to flavor and thin the sauces. For a thinner sauce, add the nectar a tablespoon at a time until the sauces are the desired consistency. To use the sauces to create a heart pattern, spoon or squeeze solid circles of raspberry mixture onto the mango mixture. Make up to eight circles in a row, leaving about ¼ inch between them. Using a toothpick or the tip of a sharp knife, draw a straight line through the middle of the circles for a pretty string of hearts.

Cook's Tip on Leftover Nectar

Combine equal amounts of nectar and club soda or sparkling water. Pour over ice, garnish with fresh fruit, and enjoy.

(PER SERVING)

Calories 53
Protein 0 g
Carbohydrates 14 g
Cholesterol 0 mg
Total Fat 0 g
  Saturated 0 g
  Polyunsaturated 0 g
  Monounsaturated 0 g
Fiber 2 g
Sodium 1 mg

Cheesecake Sauce

■ Serves 16; 2 tablespoons per serving
■ Preparation time: 5 minutes

This versatile sauce will come in handy to serve with assorted fruit or on carrot cake muffins or angel food cake.

8-ounce tub nonfat or low-fat cream cheese (1 cup)

8-ounce container fat-free or low-fat vanilla yogurt (1 cup)

⅔ cup unsifted confectioners' sugar

¾ teaspoon vanilla extract

In a food processor or blender, process all ingredients until completely smooth.

Serve immediately or cover with plastic wrap and refrigerate until needed.

(PER SERVING)

Calories 42

Protein 7 g

Carbohydrates 8 g

Cholesterol 2 mg

Total Fat 0 g

  Saturated 0 g

  Polyunsaturated 0 g

  Monounsaturated 0 g

Fiber 0 g

Sodium 94 mg

Apricot Dessert Sauce

Serves 10; 2 tablespoons per serving ■
Preparation time: 5 minutes ■

Whether you serve it over angel food cake, reduced-fat pound cake, or fresh fruit, this sauce is as delightful as it is unusual.

½ cup fat-free or low-fat vanilla yogurt

½ cup all-fruit apricot spread

1 teaspoon vanilla extract

½ teaspoon curry powder (optional)

½ cup fat-free or low-fat vanilla yogurt

½ cup frozen fat-free or light whipped topping, thawed

In a small mixing bowl, whisk together ½ cup yogurt, apricot spread, vanilla, and curry powder until smooth.

Fold in remaining ingredients. Serve immediately or cover with plastic wrap and refrigerate until needed.

COOK'S TIP

Serve sauce the same day it is made for peak flavors.

(PER SERVING)

Calories 54

Protein 1 g

Carbohydrates 12 g

Cholesterol 0 mg

Total Fat 0 g

  Saturated 0 g

  Polyunsaturated 0 g

  Monounsaturated 0 g

Fiber 0 g

Sodium 17 mg

American Heart Association Operating Units and Affiliates

For further information about American Heart Association programs and services, call 1-800-AHA-USA1 (1-800-242-8721) or contact us online at http://www.americanheart.org. For information about the American Stroke Association, a division of the American Heart Association, call 1-888-4STROKE (1-888-478-7653).

NATIONAL CENTER
American Heart Association
7272 Greenville Avenue
Dallas, TX 75231-4596
214-373-6300

OPERATING UNITS OF NATIONAL CENTER
Office of Public Advocacy
Washington, DC

American Heart Association, Hawaii
Honolulu, HI

AFFILIATES
Desert/Mountain Affiliate
Arizona, Colorado, New Mexico, Wyoming
Denver, CO

Florida/Puerto Rico Affiliate
St. Petersburg, FL

Heartland Affiliate
Arkansas, Iowa, Kansas, Missouri, Nebraska, Oklahoma
Topeka, KS

Heritage Affiliate
Connecticut, New Jersey, New York City, Long Island
New York, NY

Mid-Atlantic Affiliate
Maryland, Nation's Capital, North Carolina, South Carolina, Virginia
Glen Allen, VA

Midwest Affiliate
Illinois, Indiana, Michigan
Chicago, IL

New England Affiliate
Maine, Massachusetts, New Hampshire, Rhode Island, Vermont
Framingham, MA

New York State Affiliate
Syracuse, NY

Northland Affiliate
Minnesota, North Dakota, South Dakota, Wisconsin
Minneapolis, MN

Northwest Affiliate
Alaska, Idaho, Montana, Oregon, Washington
Seattle, WA

Ohio Valley Affiliate
Kentucky, Ohio, West Virginia
Columbus, OH

Pennsylvania Delaware Affiliate
Delaware, Pennsylvania
Wormleysburg, PA

Southeast Affiliate
Alabama, Georgia, Louisiana, Mississippi, Tennessee
Marietta, GA

Texas Affiliate
Austin, TX

Western States Affiliate
California, Nevada, Utah
Los Angeles, CA

Index

A

acceptable fats:
in food pyramid, 10
in recipes, 28–29
acceptable margarine, 28
acceptable vegetable oil, 28–29
acorn squash:
Orange-Flavored Acorn Squash
and Sweet Potato, 283
adzuki beans:
Adzuki Beans and Rice, 246–47
cook's tip on, 247
alcohol, 8
All-in-One recipes, 14
Adzuki Beans and Rice, 246–7
Beef with Barley and Vegetables,
206
Beef with Rice Noodles and
Vegetables, 191
Bell Pepper Chicken and Noodles,
164
Blackberry-Glazed Pork with
Mixed Rice and Broccoli, 220
Bloody Mary Chicken and Rice,
162
Blue Cheese Beef and Fries, 200
Brown Rice and Quinoa Pilaf,
244
Burgundy Beef Stew, 190
Butter Bean, Chicken, and
Vegetable Stew, 158
Cajun Skillet Supper, 210
Cheddar Jack Chili Mac, 209
Chicken Fajita Pasta with Chipotle
Alfredo Sauce, 165
Chicken, Pasta, and Vegetable
Casserole, 173
Chicken, Spinach, and Pasta
Casserole, 152–3
Chili-Style Beef Stew, 201
Cook's-Choice Fried Rice, 216

Curried Chicken, Pasta, and
Vegetable Casserole, 172
Curried Pasta and Vegetable
Casserole, 172
Dilled Chicken with Mushrooms
and Rice, 163
Exotic Mushroom Stroganoff, 240
Farmer's Market Stovetop
Casserole, 255
French Turkey Stew, 227
French Veal Stew, 226–7
Gnocchi with Italian Turkey
Sausage and Vegetables, 261
Green Chile, Black Bean, and
Corn Stew, 247
Grilled Tuna Niçoise, 128
Ham and Vegetable Casserole, 221
Italian Gnocchi with Vegetables,
260–61
Mushroom-Spinach Stroganoff,
240–1
No-Chop Stew, 207
Oven-Roasted Vegetables and
Pasta, 236
Pasta with Kale and Sun-Dried
Tomatoes, 242
Pasta and Vegetable Casserole, 173
Red-Hot Chicken Stir-Fry, 215
Red-Hot Pork Stir-Fry, 214
Red Lentils with Vegetables and
Brown Rice, 253
Rigatoni with Cauliflower and
Tomato Sauce, 238
Roast Beef with Baby Carrots,
Onions, and Potatoes, 198–9
Rosemary Peas and Pasta, 237
Slow-Cooker Chicken and Bell
Pepper Stew, 145
Smoked Sausage Skillet Supper, 224
Southwestern Posole Stew, 254
Spinach Stroganoff, 241

Green Chile, Black Bean, and
Corn Stew, 249
Italian Bean and Tuna Salad, 81
Italian Bean Stew with Turkey and
Ham, 180
mashed, cook's tip on, 103
Mexican Bean Dip, 38
Mixed Bean and Pasta Soup, 61
in Vegetarian Taco Salad, 89
White Bean and Pasta Soup, 61
beef, 185–227
Beef and Caramelized Onion on
Hot French Bread, 104
Beef Salad with Horseradish
Dressing, 86–87
Beef Salad with Vinaigrette
Dressing, 86–87
Beef Strips with Caramelized
Onions and Mashed Potatoes,
192
Beef Tenderloin with Mixed Baby
Greens, 194–95
Beef with Barley and Vegetables,
206
Beef with Rice Noodles and
Vegetables, 191
Blue Cheese Beef and Fries, 200
Burgundy Beef Stew, 190
Cajun Skillet Supper, 210
Cheddar Jack Chili Mac, 209
Chili-Style Beef Stew, 201
cook's tip on yield of, 87
Flank Steak Burritos, 103
Glazed Beef Strips with Sugar
Snap Peas, 188
Grilled Sirloin with Honey
Mustard Marinade, 187
Ground Beef and Shredded Potato
Casserole, 204–5
lean, cook's tip on, 199
Meatball Soup with Sun-Dried
Tomatoes and Swiss Chard,
58–59
Mediterranean Beef and Rice, 208
Mixed Kebabs, 140–41
No-Chop Stew, 207
Picante Meat Loaf with Baked
Potatoes, 202
Roast Beef with Baby Carrots,
Onions, and Potatoes, 198–99

Taco-Rubbed Flank Steak, 193
Tex-Mex Rice and Meatballs, 203
Thai Beef Salad, 88
Tuscan Braised Beef, 196–97
beef broth, cook's tip on, 210
bell pepper(s):
Bell Pepper Chicken and Noodles,
164
Bell Peppers with Nuts and Olives,
278
Cheese-Filled Bell Pepper Boats,
40
Roasted Red Bell Pepper Dressing,
95
Slow-Cooker Chicken and Bell
Pepper Stew, 145
berry(ies):
cook's tip on thawing of, 293
freezing tips for, 24
Heavenly Frozen Angel Food and
Berry Pie, 308
see also specific berries
beta carotene, 11
beverages, 36
leftover nectar in, 319
Morning Energy Drink, 47
Orange Shakes, 48
Pineapple Shakes, 48
Strawberry Mint Smoothie, 49
Strawberry Mint Spritzer, 49
water, 10
black bean(s):
Black Bean and Rice Salad, 248
Black Beans and Rice, 248
Green Chile, Black Bean, and
Corn Stew, 249
blackberry(ies):
Blackberry-Glazed Pork with
Mixed Rice and Broccoli, 220
Heavenly Frozen Angel Food and
Berry Pie, 308
Peach Fans on Blackberry-Lime
Sauce, 74
black-eyed peas:
Sweet-and-Sour Black-Eyed Peas
with Ham, 222
Black-Peppered Corn, 274
blood pressure claims, food labels
and, 21
Bloody Mary Chicken and Rice, 162

blueberry(ies):
  cook's tip on thawing of, 293
  Lemony Blueberry Coffeecake,
    290–91
  Yogurt Brûlée with Blueberries, 293
Blue Cheese Beef and Fries, 200
boiling, tips on, 32, 91
bok choy:
  cook's tip on, 115
  Orange Roughy with Bok Choy
    and Cherry Tomatoes, 114–15
Bourbon Sauce, 312–13
braising, 25–26
Bread Pudding with Peaches and
    Bourbon Sauce, 312–13
breads, 287–92
  Cinnamon Sticks, 289
  cook's tip on flour, 291
  in food pyramid, 9
  Garlic Toasts, 194
  Herb Sticks, 289
  Lemony Blueberry Coffeecake,
    290–91
  Mini Cinnamon Stackups, 292
  Raspberry Coffeecake, 291
  shopping tips for, 17–18
  see also sandwiches
breakfast dishes, 289–95
  Cinnamon Sticks, 289
  Fruitful Brown Rice Cereal, 294
  Huevos Rancheros Casserole, 295
  Lemony Blueberry Coffeecake,
    290–91
  Mini Cinnamon Stackups, 292
  Morning Energy Drink, 47
  Morning Energy "Soup," 47
  Raspberry Coffeecake, 291
  Yogurt Brûlée with Blueberries,
    293
broccoli:
  Blackberry-Glazed Pork with
    Mixed Rice and Broccoli, 220
  Broccoli Potato Frittata, 256
  Broccoli with Sweet-and-Sour
    Tangerine Sauce, 270
  Sesame Broccoli, 271
  Tuna Casserole with Broccoli and
    Water Chestnuts, 129
  Turkey and Broccoli Stir-Fry,
    176–77

broiling, 25
  cook's tip on timing of, 193
  see also grilling
broth, freezer tips for, 23
brown rice:
  Brown Rice and Quinoa Pilaf, 244
  Fruitful Brown Rice Cereal, 294
  Red Lentils with Vegetables and
    Brown Rice, 253
brûlée:
  Yogurt Brûlée with Blueberries,
    293
brussels sprouts:
  Curried Brussels Sprouts, 272
bulgur:
  Bulgur-Stuffed Crookneck Squash,
    284–85
  cook's tip on, 251
burgers:
  Bean and Vegetable Burgers, 250
Burgundy Beef Stew, 190
burritos:
  Flank Steak Burritos, 103
butcher, services of, 32
butter, saturated fat in, 6
butter bean(s):
  Butter Bean, Chicken, and
    Vegetable Stew, 158
  cook's tip on, 158
butternut squash:
  Butternut Squash Soup, 53
  frozen, cook's tip on, 53
  with mashed potatoes, 53

C

cabbage:
  Cabbage Slaw with Roasted
    Peanut Oil Dressing, 72
  Chinese, cook's tip on, 71
  Warm Napa Slaw, 70–71
  Warm Napa Slaw with Chicken,
    70–71
cacciatore:
  Tofu Cacciatore, 239
Cajun Baked Fish, 132–33
Cajun Frittata with Pasta, 258–59
Cajun Skillet Supper, 210

chicken (cont'd):
cook's tips on, 149, 169
Corn and Chicken Chowder, 55
Creamed Chicken and Vegetables,
175
Crispy Chicken with Creamy
Gravy, 146
Curried Chicken, Pasta, and
Vegetable Casserole, 172–73
Curried Chicken and Cauliflower,
157
Curried Pasta and Vegetable
Casserole, 172
Dilled Chicken with Mushrooms
and Rice, 163
disposable plastic gloves for use
with, 169
Far East Chicken Salad, 93
in food pyramid, 9
freezing tips for, 24, 32
Greek Chicken Thighs, 166
Grilled Chicken with Green Chiles
and Cheese, 154–55
Italian Grilled Chicken, 154–55
Italian Stir-Fry, 161
Lemongrass Chicken with Snow
Peas and Jasmine Rice, 174
Mediterranean Chicken in a Slow
Cooker, 167
Mixed Kebabs, 140–41
Orange-Barbecue Chicken
Chunks, 150
Polynesian Chicken in a Slow
Cooker, 167
Red-Hot Chicken Stir-Fry, 215
Roasted Chicken Breasts with
Garlic Gravy, 147
shopping tips for, 16
Slow-Cooker Chicken and Bell
Pepper Stew, 145
Sour Cream Chicken Enchiladas,
170–71
Southwestern Chicken Salad,
82–83
Southwestern-Style Roasted
Chicken, 168–69
Spicy Honey-Kissed Chicken, 151
Sun-Dried Tomato Pesto Chicken
and Pasta, 148–49

time-saver for, 83
Two-Way Border Chicken, 156
Warm Napa Slaw with Chicken,
70–71
white meat, cook's tip on, 149
yields of, 169
chick-peas:
Curried Lamb Stew with Chick-
Peas, 225
chile peppers:
cook's tip on, 77
Green Chile, Black Bean, and
Corn Stew, 249
Grilled Chicken with Green Chiles
and Cheese, 154–55
chili:
Chili-Style Beef Stew, 201
Vegetarian Chili, 251
Chilled Strawberry Orange Soup, 63
Chinese cabbage, cook's tip on, 71
chipotle sauce:
Chicken Fajita Pasta with Chipotle
Alfredo Sauce, 165
chocolate:
Chocolate Almond Angel Food
Cake with Oranges, 301
Chocolate Hazelnut Angel Food
Cake with Bananas, 300–302
Chocolate Pistachio Angel Food
Cake with Strawberries, 302
Chocolate Pudding Cake, 299
Chocolate Walnut Angel Food
Cake with Raspberries, 301
Devil's Food Cake with Caramel
Drizzles, 303
in Frozen Dessert Terrine, 317
cholesterol, 6, 7, 11, 21
chowder:
Corn and Cheddar Chowder, 55
Corn and Chicken Chowder, 55
Chunky Creole Sauce, 134
cinnamon:
Cinnamon Apple Bars, 311
Cinnamon Sticks, 289
Cinnamon Sugar Phyllo Snacks,
43
Cranberry Cinnamon Baked
Apples, 315
Mini Cinnamon Stackups, 292

coring and seeding tomatoes, cook's
tip on, 118
corn:
Black-Peppered Corn, 274
Corn and Cheddar Chowder, 55
Corn and Chicken Chowder, 55
Green Chile, Black Bean, and
Corn Stew, 249
couscous:
Fresh Herb Couscous Salad, 90
cranberry:
Cranberry and Cream Cheese
Turkey Sandwiches, 102
Cranberry Cinnamon Baked
Apples, 315
Turkey Breast with Cranberry Sage
Stuffing, 182
cream cheese:
Cranberry and Cream Cheese
Turkey Sandwiches, 102
Creamed Chicken and Vegetables,
175
Creamed Peas, 282
Creamed Spinach, 282
Creamed Tuna and Vegetables, 175
Creamy Mushroom Barley Soup, 62
crisp:
Apple Crisp, 309
Pear Crisp, 309
Crispy Chicken with Creamy Gravy,
146
crookneck squash:
Bulgur-Stuffed Crookneck Squash,
284–85
Crumb-Crusted Fish Fillets, 132–33
cucumber(s):
English, cook's tip on, 72
Greek Cucumber Salad, 73
cupcakes:
Lemon Cupcakes with Apricot
Glaze, 305
Curried Brussels Sprouts, 272
Curried Chicken, Pasta, and
Vegetable Casserole, 172–73
Curried Chicken and Cauliflower,
157
Curried Lamb Stew with Chick-Peas,
225
Curried Pasta and Vegetable
Casserole, 172

D

dairy products:
in food pyramid, 9
shopping tips for, 16–17
deglazing, cook's tip on, 195
desserts, 297–322
Ambrosia Parfait, 314
Apple Crisp, 309
Apricot Dessert Sauce, 321
Bread Pudding with Peaches and
Bourbon Sauce, 312–13
Cheesecake Sauce, 320
Chocolate Almond Angel Food
Cake with Oranges, 301
Chocolate Hazelnut Angel Food
Cake with Bananas, 300–302
Chocolate Pistachio Angel Food
Cake with Strawberries, 302
Chocolate Pudding Cake, 299
Chocolate Walnut Angel Food
Cake with Raspberries, 301
Cinnamon Apple Bars, 311
Cranberry Cinnamon Baked
Apples, 315
Devil's Food Cake with Caramel
Drizzles, 303
flavored syrups, cook's tip on,
302
Frozen Dessert Terrine, 317
Ginger Banana Snacks, 310
Ginger Snacks, 310
Heavenly Frozen Angel Food and
Berry Pie, 308
Lemon Cake with Apricot Glaze,
304–5
Lemon Cake with Apricot
Topping, 304
Lemon Cupcakes with Apricot
Glaze, 305
Mango and Raspberry Fruit
Sauces, 318–19
Nectarine and Raspberry Pie with
Phyllo Crust, 306–7
nectar, cook's tip on leftover,
319
Pear Crisp, 309
phyllo, cook's tip on, 307
Pineapple Shakes, frozen variation,
48

fish sauce, cook's tip on, 88
flank steak:
  Flank Steak Burritos, 103
  Taco-Rubbed Flank Steak, 193
flavored syrups, cook's tip on, 302
flour, cook's tip on, 291
food certification, American Heart
    Association program of, 21
food labels, 19–21
food preparation, organization of,
    22–24
food processors, 31
food pyramid, 8–9
free radicals, 11
freezer basics, 23–24, 32
freezing liquids, cook's tip on, 316
French Turkey Stew, 227
French Veal Stew, 226–27
Fresh Herb Couscous Salad, 90
fried rice:
  Cook's-Choice Fried Rice, 216
  cook's tip on, 216
fries:
  Blue Cheese Beef and Fries, 200
frittatas:
  Broccoli Potato Frittata, 256
  Cajun Frittata with Pasta, 258–59
  Pasta Frittata, 258–59
  Spanish Tortilla, 257
frozen desserts:
  Frozen Dessert Terrine, 317
  Heavenly Frozen Angel Food and
    Berry Pie, 308
  Pineapple Shakes variation, 48
  Two-Way Mixed-Fruit Freeze, 316
  Two-Way Strawberry Freeze, 316
fruit(s):
  Ambrosia Parfait, 314
  food labels and, 21
  in food pyramid, 9
  freezing juice of, 23–24
  Fruitful Brown Rice Cereal, 294
  Mixed Fruit Salad with Mango
    Dressing, 76
  Mixed Salad Greens and Fruit
    with Fresh Strawberry
    Vinaigrette, 67
  nectar, cook's tip on leftover,
    319
  shopping tips for, 17

Two-Way Mixed-Fruit Freeze,
    316
  see also specific fruits

G

garlic:
  cook's tip on, 45
  Garlic Toasts, 194
  Grilled Tuna with Garlic, 126
  Roasted Chicken Breasts with
    Garlic Gravy, 147
gelatin salads:
  Lime-Pineapple Gelatin Salad, 78
  Orange-Pineapple Gelatin Salad,
    78
German Potato Salad, 79
Ginger Banana Snacks, 310
Ginger Snacks, 310
glazes:
  deglazing, cook's tip on, 195
  Devil's Food Cake with Caramel
    Drizzles, 303
  Glazed Beef Strips with Sugar
    Snap Peas, 188
  Lemon Cake with Apricot Glaze,
    304–5
  Lemon Cupcakes with Apricot
    Glaze, 305
  Maple-Glazed Carrots, 273
gloves, disposable, uses for, 169
gnocchi:
  cook's tip on, 261
  Gnocchi with Italian Turkey
    Sausage and Vegetables, 261
  Italian Gnocchi with Vegetables,
    260–61
goat cheese:
  Pear and Goat Cheese Salad, 75
  Tomato, Oregano, and Goat
    Cheese Sandwiches, 105
grains:
  food labels and claims about, 21
  in food pyramid, 9
  shopping tips for, 17–18
  see also specific grains
grapefruit:
  Chicken and Grapefruit Salad, 85
  see also citrus fruits

gravy:
    Crispy Chicken with Creamy
        Gravy, 146
    fat-free, cook's tip on, 200
    Roasted Chicken Breasts with
        Garlic Gravy, 147
Greek Chicken Thighs, 166
Greek Cucumber Salad, 73
Greek Green Beans, 275
Greek White Beans, 252
Green and Petite Pea Salad with
    Feta, 68
green beans:
    Greek Green Beans, 275
green chile(s):
    Green Chile, Black Bean, and
        Corn Stew, 249
    Grilled Chicken with Green Chiles
        and Cheese, 154–55
greens:
    Beef Tenderloin with Mixed Baby
        Greens, 194–95
    Mixed Salad Greens and Fruit
        with Fresh Strawberry
        Vinaigrette, 67
    Portobello Pizza with Peppery
        Greens, 231
    premixed packages of, 67
    see also salads
grilling, 25
    Barbecued Chicken Dijon, 155
    Barbecue Shrimp Kebabs, 137
    cook's tip on timing of, 193
    Grilled Chicken with Green Chiles
        and Cheese, 154–55
    Grilled Sirloin with Honey
        Mustard Marinade, 187
    Grilled Tuna Niçoise, 128
    Grilled Tuna with Garlic, 126
    Grilled Turkey Cutlets with
        Pineapple, 181
    Italian Grilled Chicken,
        154–55
    Mixed Kebabs, 140–41
ground beef:
    Beef with Barley and Vegetables,
        206
    Cajun Skillet Supper, 210
    Cheddar Jack Chili Mac, 209

Ground Beef and Shredded Potato
    Casserole, 204–5
Meatball Soup with Sun-Dried
    Tomatoes and Swiss Chard,
    58–59
Mediterranean Beef and Rice,
    208
No-Chop Stew, 207
Picante Meat Loaf with Baked
    Potatoes, 202
Tex-Mex Rice and Meatballs, 203

H

Halibut and Vegetable Medley, 113
ham:
    Ham and Hash Brown Casserole,
        223
    Ham and Vegetable Casserole, 221
    Italian Bean Stew with Turkey and
        Ham, 180
    Sweet-and-Sour Black-Eyed Peas
        with Ham, 222
Hawaiian-Style Tuna, 127
health claims, on food labels, 21
Healthy Heart Food Pyramid, 8–9
heart disease claims, food labels and,
    21
Heavenly Frozen Angel Food and
    Berry Pie, 308
herb(s):
    Fresh Herb Couscous Salad, 90
    Herbed Peas and Mushrooms,
        277
    herbes de Provence, cook's tips on,
        123
    Herb Sticks, 289
    rubs, see rubs
    storage of, 32
    see also specific herbs
hominy:
    cook's tip on, 254
    in Southwestern Posole Stew, 254
Honey Mustard Salmon, 117
horseradish:
    Beef Salad with Horseradish
        Dressing, 86–87

hot chile peppers, cook's tip on, 77
Huevos Rancheros Casserole, 295

I

ingredients:
  flexibility in use of, 32
  tips for, 32
instant-read thermometers, cook's tip on, 197
Italian Bean and Tuna Salad, 81
Italian Bean Stew with Turkey and Ham, 180
Italian Gnocchi with Vegetables, 260–61
Italian Grilled Chicken, 154–55
Italian Marinade, 140
Italian Quiche in Phyllo Shells, 42–43
Italian Stir-Fry, 161
Italian Vegetables, 235
Italian Vegetable Stew, 234
Italian Vegetable Stew with Pasta, 235

J

jasmine rice:
  Lemongrass Chicken with Snow Peas and Jasmine Rice, 174
  Vegetables in Thai Sauce with Jasmine Rice, 243
jícama, cook's tip on, 83
juice, freezing tips for, 23–24

K

kale:
  cook's tip on, 242
  Pasta with Kale and Sun-Dried Tomatoes, 242
kebabs:
  Barbecue Shrimp Kebabs, 137
  Mixed Kebabs, 140–41

key words, on food labels, 20–21
knives, sharp, 31

L

labels, nutrition, 19–21
lamb:
  Curried Lamb Stew with Chick-Peas, 225
LDLs (low-density lipoproteins), 11
lean meat, cook's tip on, 199
leftovers:
  recipes for, 13, 14
lemon:
  Lemon Cake with Apricot Glaze, 304–5
  Lemon Cake with Apricot Topping, 304
  Lemon Cupcakes with Apricot Glaze, 305
  Lemony Blueberry Coffeecake, 290–91
  Pan-Blackened Scallops over Lemon Rice, 136
  Roasted Lemon Pork with Cinnamon Sweet Potatoes, 212
  see also citrus fruits
Lemongrass Chicken with Snow Peas and Jasmine Rice, 174
lentil(s):
  red, cook's tip on, 253
  Red Lentils with Vegetables and Brown Rice, 253
  Spinach Lentil Soup, 57
Lime-Pineapple Gelatin Salad, 78
liquids, cook's tip on freezing of, 316
low-density lipoproteins (LDLs), 11
low-sodium beef broth, cook's tip on, 210

M

mandolines, cook's tip on, 200
mango:
  Mango and Raspberry Fruit Sauces, 318–19

Portobello Sandwiches with Zesty
Red Onions, 106–7
Stacked Mushroom Nachos, 46

N

nachos:
Stacked Mushroom Nachos, 46
napa cabbage:
cook's tip on, 71
Warm Napa Slaw, 70–71
Warm Napa Slaw with Chicken,
70–71
Nectarine and Raspberry Pie with
Phyllo Crust, 306–7
nectar, cook's tip on leftover, 319
New Classic recipes, 13, 14
Barbecued Chicken Dijon, 155
Black Beans and Rice, 248
Cajun Baked Fish, 132–3
Celery-Sage Pork Chops, 218–19
Cheddar Jack Chili Mac, 209
Crispy Chicken with Creamy
Gravy, 146
Crumb-Crusted Fish Fillets,
132
Grilled Chicken with Green Chiles
and Cheese, 154
Italian Bean and Tuna Salad, 81
Italian Grilled Chicken, 154–5
Pita Pizzas, 233
Rosemary Braised Pork Chops,
218–19
Tuna Casserole with Broccoli and
Water Chestnuts, 129
Tuna Pita Melts, 99
Vegetarian Taco Salad, 89
No-Chop Stew, 207
nutrient analysis, in recipes, 28–30
nutrients, daily values for, 20
nutrition labels, 19–21

O

oils, acceptable, 28–29
omega–3 fatty acids, 10, 16

onions:
cook's tip on, 279
freezing tips for, 24
Open-Face Broiled Italian Vegetable
Sandwiches, 108
orange(s):
Chilled Strawberry Orange Soup,
63
Chocolate Almond Angel Food
Cake with Oranges, 301
Orange-Barbecue Chicken
Chunks, 150
Orange-Flavored Acorn Squash
and Sweet Potato, 283
Orange-Pineapple Gelatin Salad,
78
Orange Sesame Pork, 213
Orange Shakes, 48
see also citrus fruits
orange roughy:
cook's tip on, 133
Orange Roughy with Bok Choy
and Cherry Tomatoes, 114–15
organization, 22–24
Orzo Salad with Green Peas and
Artichokes, 91
Oven-Roasted Vegetables and Pasta,
236

P

Pan-Blackened Scallops over Lemon
Rice, 136
parfait:
Ambrosia Parfait, 314
Parmesan Pork Medallions, 211
pasta:
Basil-Parmesan Pesto Chicken and
Pasta, 148–49
Beef with Rice Noodles and
Vegetables, 191
Bell Pepper Chicken and Noodles,
164
Cajun Frittata with Pasta, 258–59
Chicken, Pasta, and Vegetable
Casserole, 173
Chicken, Spinach, and Pasta
Casserole, 152–53

V

veal:
  French Veal Stew, 226–27
vegetable(s):
  Avocado Veggie Wraps, 109
  Barley and Vegetable Salad, 80
  Bean and Vegetable Burgers, 250
  Beef with Barley and Vegetables, 206
  Beef with Rice Noodles and Vegetables, 191
  Butter Bean, Chicken, and Vegetable Stew, 158
  Chicken, Pasta, and Vegetable Casserole, 173
  Chicken and Vegetable Stir-Fry, 160–61
  Creamed Chicken and Vegetables, 175
  Creamed Tuna and Vegetables, 175
  Curried Chicken, Pasta, and Vegetable Casserole, 172–73
  Curried Pasta and Vegetable Casserole, 172
  Farmers' Market Stovetop Casserole, 255
  food labels and, 21
  in food pyramid, 9
  frozen, refreshing of, 33
  Gnocchi with Italian Turkey Sausage and Vegetables, 261
  Halibut and Vegetable Medley, 113
  Ham and Vegetable Casserole, 221
  Italian Gnocchi with Vegetables, 260–61
  Italian Vegetables, 235
  Italian Vegetable Stew, 234
  Italian Vegetable Stew with Pasta, 235
  Mini Vegetable Cheese Balls, 39
  Mozzarella Polenta with Roasted Vegetable Salsa, 262–63
  Open-Face Broiled Italian Vegetable Sandwiches, 108
  Oven-Roasted Vegetables and Pasta, 236
  Pasta and Vegetable Casserole, 173
  Pasta with Italian Vegetables, 234–35
  Red Lentils with Vegetables and Brown Rice, 253
  Roasted Vegetable Spread, 41
  shopping tips for, 17
  Sole and Vegetable Terrine, 122–23
  thawing, cook's tip on, 68
  Vegetables in Thai Sauce with Jasmine Rice, 243
  see also side dishes; vegetarian entrées; specific vegetables
vegetable oil, acceptable, 28–29
vegetarian entrées, 229–64
  Adzuki Beans and Rice, 246–47
  Bean and Vegetable Burgers, 250
  Black Bean and Rice Salad, 248
  Black Beans and Rice, 248
  Broccoli Potato Frittata, 256
  Brown Rice and Quinoa Pilaf, 244
  Exotic Mushroom Stroganoff, 240–41
  Farmers' Market Stovetop Casserole, 255
  Greek White Beans, 252
  Green Chile, Black Bean, and Corn Stew, 249
  Italian Gnocchi with Vegetables, 260–61
  Italian Vegetables, 235
  Italian Vegetable Stew, 234–35
  Italian Vegetable Stew with Pasta, 235
  Mozzarella Polenta with Roasted Vegetable Salsa, 262–63
  Mushroom Quesadillas, 264
  Mushroom-Spinach Stroganoff, 240–41
  Oven-Roasted Vegetables and Pasta, 236
  Pasta and Vegetable Casserole, 173
  Pasta Frittata, 258–59
  Pasta with Italian Vegetables, 234–35
  Pasta with Kale and Sun-Dried Tomatoes, 242
  Pita Pizzas, 233

Notes

Notes

Notes

Notes

Notes

Notes